68 Remembers

Anecdotes from Newcastle doctors who qualified in 1968.
The definitive edition.

Collated by
Peter Tate and Keith Baxby

April 2021

ISBN: 9798734520345

Introduction

Members of the Class of 68 have lived through astonishing changes in the way medicine is learned and practiced. Many pages could be filled with lists of contrasts between "Then and Now" and it is difficult to select a few examples. We spent four terms (even that... er... term has been replaced) dissecting a cadaver, memorising lists of branches, relations and innervations, well over 95% of which was never used by well over 95% of us. Almost our only other sources of information were lectures and textbooks. If someone had told us in the mid-60s that within our lifetimes students would be able to obtain any information they needed from a gadget like a minuscule television which they could carry in a pocket they would have had the Glaswegian response I recall Prof Scothorne giving to an erring classmate: "Och- awa' get yer heid examined!" We have seen practice changed beyond what we could have imagined by, for instance, successful chemotherapy for malignancies which were a death sentence when we qualified; minimally invasive surgery; changes in the management of pain, diabetes, heart disease, etc., etc; and, less dramatic but just as important, a transformation of communication with patients. Many of us have benefitted from these changes as patients ourselves. Some of the contributions to this anthology remind us of how very different our training and early practice were from what happens now.

Despite all the changes, one feature of being a doctor remains: a medical degree is a ticket for a seat in the front row at the theatre of human behaviour in its myriad manifestations. We have been privileged to have an insight into people's lives and to help them, however inadequately, at a low point in those lives. I have yet to meet a former classmate who regrets their decision to study medicine at Newcastle. Many of these contributions reflect the endless variety of human behaviour and the gratitude, enthusiasm and pleasure, as well as the heartache, brought by doctoring in its many forms. We have been a very fortunate generation and many of us feel that "we had the best of it", not envying our successors, especially at this time of writing.

At the start of Lockdown One, Stuart Walton and John Davies invited those of the Class who were interested to form a WhatsApp group so we could brighten the gloom by sharing jokes, cartoons, reminiscences and much else. With the approach of Christmas 2020 I suggested that most of us would have an anecdote from our careers which we could share with the group to further cheer us up. Peter Tate, who has published several books (and who has been a prime mover in the transformation of communication referred to above) quickly offered to turn any contributions into an anthology, using his editing and publishing experience. He has cajoled, collated and crafted to produce what you have here. We are grateful to all contributors, and to all who have bought the anthology in support of charity; we hope you enjoy it.

Keith Baxby
Dundee,
21 January 2021.

The stories kept on coming, so here are the definitive memories of the year of 68. It is a really good read.
All monies received goes to the Newcastle University Covid-19 Emergency Fund for Students.

Peter Tate
Poundbury
Dorchester
peter.spud@gmail.com

April 8th, 2021.

All contributions, as our year was structured, are in alphabetical order. 30 in total.

Malcolm Ayre

Two memorable cases

My first job after qualifying was as a surgical H.O. at Sunderland Royal infirmary. The Royal was the only hospital in the Sunderland group with a casualty department, so all acute cases, major and minor, were seen there first. Part of my job was to be on call for casualty every night I was on duty to take any surgical admissions that could not be transferred to the appropriate hospital in the group which was admitting that night.

I recall two memorable cases. One was a middle aged, overweight, and very drunk lady who had been involved in an R.T.A. crossing from the pub to the bus stop; she had been run over by a scooter, and her right lower leg was so severely injured it needed amputation All the way through assessment she was singing and unable to give a proper history; the alcohol was doing a good job as an analgesic. When told that she was going to lose her leg, she changed to a rendition of Sinatra's "All of me, why not take all of me" and continued singing this all the way to the ward.

The second patient was a young man in his 20's with a suspected perforated peptic ulcer. Out drinking with his friends, he suddenly doubled over with severe upper abdominal pain. Assessed by the SHO he was waiting for a plain X ray abdomen and I was instructed to give him an injection of I.V. probanthine in the belief it would reduce acid secretion. I had just finished when he suddenly sat up and said "Eee, that's smashin Doc, pains gone", and swung his legs over the edge of the couch. When instructed to lie down as he needed further tests, he said "I'm fine now and me mates are waiting for me, it's only 9 o'clock and there's plenty of drinking time left". He set off, out through the door with sister shouting that he needed to sign himself out against medical advice, and the porter chasing after him. That was the last we saw of him, so the presumptive diagnosis was undoubtedly wrong.

This was the real side of medicine, the human side of, the bit we weren't taught because you had to learn it through experience, the humorous and the tragic incidents that were to make up the rest of our working lives.

Keith Baxby

An elective in Ulster

Thanks to the skills of John Davies, I can submit this digitised B&W version of a 2x2 colour slide (remember those?). The photo was taken in July 1966 atop Slieve Donard, the highest mountain in Ulster, when we were doing our elective period in Downpatrick.

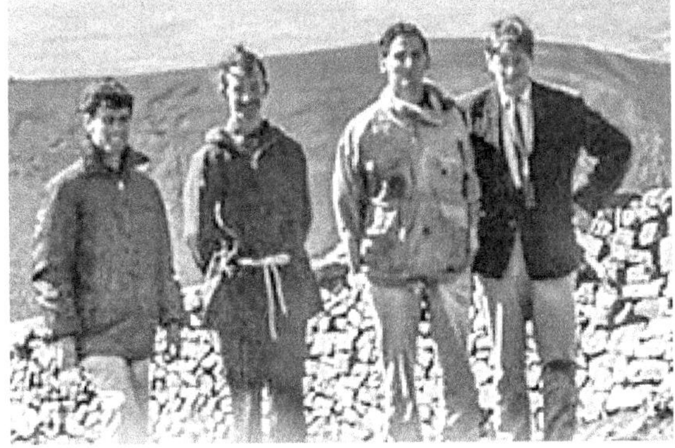

On the left is Graeme Oliver. Second right is the late and much missed Iain Mungall. The idiot on the far right, wearing a corduroy blazer, white shirt and tie (well, somebody had to maintain standards) is myself. Slieve Donard is 850 metres high, so the weather must have been good- or perhaps it was just that I had left all my proper kit, left over from a trip to the Alps a year earlier, back at home.

The character - and I mean character - second left is Tommy Bingham, a psychiatric male nurse or, to use his own term, "a keeper" from the Down and Downshire Psychiatric Hospital, where we were billeted. He had latched onto us and took a friendly concern in our welfare, including giving tips for good candidates among the nursing staff for a spot of what Tony Reed elsewhere refers to as "horizontal counselling". He had two hobbies; one, an essential for any Irishman, was "The Horses" and, as he was handsome and charismatic, the other was what he referred to as "Playing the old Irish Flute". I need not elaborate.

Although billeted at the psychiatric hospital we worked at the tiny Downpatrick Hospital which had 48 beds. There was a single houseman, Lance, who was from Tobago and also had two hobbies: cricket and sleeping.

Despite the small size, and probably because of the free accommodation and food, the hospital was very popular with students for electives.

As well as Graeme, Iain, David Fieldhouse and myself, who I think we were all billeted at the psychiatric hospital, a large bungalow in the grounds of the general hospital accommodated several other students including two Greek female students. One other was from Belfast and was preparing for his Nth resit of finals, this still being the time in Ulster when as long as you could pay the fees, you could sit the exams as many times as necessary.

There were three Edinburgh students, one being a "Wee Free", a MacDonald from Lewis. There was a piano in the residence lounge. One Sunday morning someone began to play. He had hardly played two bars when MacDonald stormed out of his room, threw open the lounge door and delivered a 17th century fire-and-brimstone sermon about the pianist putting his eternal soul in peril by desecrating the Lord's Day. This was so bizarre that I though he must be joking. I burst out laughing. He had been deadly serious, and relations were frosty for the remaining weeks.

I experienced this belief almost forty years later. I stayed in a B&B on North Uist. I was to leave on a Sunday and was asked to pay on the Saturday as handling money on a Sunday was forbidden. In the Wee Free northern half of the Western Isles Sunday is sacrosanct and nothing can be done except go to church. A lad kicking a football would be ostracised. There was a dreadful row recently when CalMac ferries wanted to land on a Sunday. A consultant colleague from a croft on Lewis told me it was actually true that the cockerel would be caught on Saturday evening and have an inverted open-weave basket placed over him until Monday morning to keep him away from the hens; avian intercourse being yet another desecration of the Sabbath. In the Catholic southern half Sunday is a day for celebration, family gatherings, music and generally putting one's eternal soul in peril by committing the ultimate Presbyterian sin: having a good time. And I guess the roosters have a better life too.

Back at the psychiatric hospital I learned that it had recently changed its name. The crockery, cutlery and linen was all marked D.L.A. This stood for "Downshire Lunatic Asylum" which it had until quite recently been called. Perhaps some things have improved.

We were in Ulster a couple of years before "The Troubles" began. I had flown from Manchester to Belfast. A contact had arranged some pigeon shooting so I took my shotgun. I checked in with it over one shoulder in a thin canvas slip. I asked what I should do with it. The check-in girl said,
"By rights firearms should go in the hold but the gun could get damaged, so just take it into the cabin and keep it under your seat".
So, I went through the departure lounge (it is hard to imagine now, but there was no scanning or security of any kind in those happier days) and up the aircraft steps. The hostess at the top had no reaction and just indicated my seat. Can you imagine what would happen now if someone checked in for a flight to Belfast with a shotgun over one shoulder?
My last memory involves the regrettably late and also much missed Howard Young. He spent his elective at a psychiatric hospital in Belfast itself. On our return to Newcastle, he had an accent that would have made Ian Paisley sound like a BBC announcer. I told him that in Downpatrick I had developed glandular fever, had been given ampicillin for the "tonsillitis" and come out in a spectacular rash. He told me he had had the same experience, and we agreed that if we found a third person, we would write it up as an eponymous syndrome. We never did, and so missed our chance of fame when the phenomenon was later recognised as being virtually a diagnostic test.

Two cases of "Renal Colic"
It has been written that each doctor has their own private cemetery, which they must visit at intervals throughout their lives. In my experience these visits, like 1970s kidney transplants, always happen in the small hours as a substitute for sleep; and the visits become more troublesome as time passes and one's own one-way trip nears. I am thankful that my cemetery, by luck rather than anything else, has very few occupants indeed; but the first took up residence only a few months after I graduated.
During one of my 24 -hour stints in Medical Cabin at the RVI a 60 year old man was sent in late in the evening with "left renal colic": in office hours he would have gone to Surgical Cabin to be seen by a surgical registrar, not a JHO "fresh from Clotho's spindle".

The pain was not classical, but Mr Feggetter had taught me that textbook presentations rarely happened in real life, and one should be suspicious when they did.
The patient was pale and clammy, as renal colic makes people. His abdomen was massive and examination meaningless, but he clearly needed an IVP. I gave him pethidine for his pain and sent him to the X-Ray department, where he died from his leaking aortic aneurysm.
I subsequently learned that people who get kidney stones usually first present in their 20s or 30s and drummed into my trainees that if someone presented with their first attack of "renal colic" in middle or later life one should be very cautious indeed.
I have tried to console myself during my visits with the thought that his chances of surviving surgery for ruptured AAA in 1969 were exceedingly small; a manoeuvre accurately described by a colleague discussing his own cemetery visits as "an intellectual and emotional cop-out".
My second "renal colic" also had an outcome which left me unhappy, but no-one died. A man in his 20s came in, rolling around with severe pain. Between gasps he gave a textbook description of renal colic. He said that he had had several kidney stones, that he knew he would need an IVP but begged for some pain relief first, with the caveat. "That pethidine stuff does not work for me, it has to be morphine". I obliged with a small IV dose. I have given enough clues for you to guess what happened next.
Within seconds of my withdrawing the needle he gave a big smile, jumped off the couch, said "Thanks Doc - that's what I needed" and ran out of the department. I wrote above that nobody died. For a few seconds I wanted to run after him and produce a different outcome but thought it might be a bad career move.
These were my first two post-graduation cases of "renal colic". I am glad they did not put me off urology for good.

Mr Hugh Brown
Some classmates will remember Hugh Brown, plastic surgeon. When I was RSO in Casualty in the RVI in 1972 he was consultant in charge of Casualty. There were no A&E consultants as such in those days, and the department was put in the charge of the most recently appointed consultant in a relevant speciality.

My first piece is not an anecdote from my experience, but I feel able to include it because it was Mr Brown's favourite joke. He told it to me in 1972 and I overheard him telling it to a retired GP at the D&NMGA visit to Howick Hall forty-three years later, so it has stood the test of time. It concerns a vet disturbed in the night by a phone call, so many of us will empathise with that. Whether any of us can empathise with the ending is another matter.

The vet is in bed; it is nearly midnight when the phone rings. He curses and picks it up. A voice says, "Is that you vet 'nary?" and he recognises the voice of his most troublesome client, an officious lady who has two Pekingese dogs.

" Yes Mrs. Johnson, how can I help?"

"Well, it is very embarrassing – you know I have two small doggies, a boy doggie and a girl doggie?"

"Yes."

"Well, they have been, you know, er, doing it and are stuck together- I cannot get them apart. You need to come here at once and separate them."

"Oh, I don't need to go to your house, we can do this over the telephone. Put your phone back on the hook, pick up the two doggies, stuck together, bring them to the phone and I will phone them up".

"That is ridiculous: what in heaven's name makes you think that phoning them up will get them apart?"

"Well," says the vet "It just worked for me!"

I recall two reasons to be grateful to Mr Brown. For the first, as RSO I got a letter from Gateshead solicitors asking me for an account of the injuries suffered by their client in an assault. I wrote back saying that I would need a signed mandate from their client, authorising me to reveal his medical details. Every classmate will agree that is normal practice. By return I got an angry response saying they "found your attitude extraordinary: surely it can be assumed that as he is our client, we have his permission to be told his medical details.

Please supply the report without further delay." Still no mandate. I was upset by this, feeling that I had acted in accordance with MDU advice and been berated for acting properly. I showed the letter to Mr Brown who offered to reply for me in his position as Consultant in Charge.

He wrote them a real stinker, starting with pointing out that I had no way of knowing that they were acting for this man; they might well be the “other side" on a fishing expedition, then pointing out that I was acting in accordance with standard medico- legal practice, and ending with his surprise that, as supposedly competent lawyers, they were unaware of the correct procedure. The mandate arrived swiftly, but no apology came.

For the second, I had the X-ray of a neck which I was unsure about. Mr Brown was dictating in the room which doubled as the coffee room and an office. I knocked on the door, film in hand and on entry moved towards the window with a view to holding the X Ray to the window, at the same time asking if he could “Take a quick look at this X-ray".

I was taken aback by his firm response of “No, I shall not". After a pause he added" But if you take it into Surgical Cabin and put it on an X-ray viewer, I shall be glad to have a proper look at it when I have finished this letter”. After he had pronounced the X-ray to be normal, he formally and firmly advised me “Never examine an X-ray by holding it against the window, and even on an X-ray viewer never “take a quick look": always examine all parts of it, methodically”.

That advice stood me in good stead. I can think off-hand of three people who are still probably walking around today thanks to his advice, which I later drummed into my own trainees.

The importance of communication

As registrar in urology at NGH in 1971 I admitted a man of 93 from Scots Gap, with retention of urine. He had all his mental faculties, and I enjoyed his account of fighting in the Boer War seventy years earlier, although even after nine years in Newcastle I found his very broad mid-Northumberland accent tricky.

He was catheterised and like all catheterised patients in those days he had daily “Catheter Toilet”. This involved a nurse retracting the prepuce (when present) with one hand and swabbing the external urethral meatus, corona and coronal sulcus with a Savlon-soaked swab with the other. A few days after admission he became very confused and was put in a side- room (which probably further increased his confusion).

On the day in question, I was on a full-dress formal ward round with Mr Yeates and the whole team.

We were some way from the side-room when I noticed a staff nurse, who was remarkably prim and strait-laced for one in her role, go into this man's side-room bearing the catheter toilet tray.
We later learned that because he was so very confused, she had seen no point in trying to explain the procedure to him, merely turned back the bedclothes, seized his *membrum virile* in her left hand and used the Savlon swab with her right. But all we had at the time was a very loud shout from the side-room "Norse, have ye got nothin' bettor to dee than play with an old man's cock?" Despite the decibel value of the shout, Mr Yeates and Sister pretended not to hear it. My attempts to keep a straight face caused a laceration inside my lower lip which hurt for days.

Three phallic problems

Many years ago, the BMJ had a paper in its Christmas edition showing that presentations do run in threes: admit two MIs, fractured necks of femur etc and a third will quickly come along more frequently than chance dictates. As SR in urology at NGH I dealt with three phallic problems in as many weeks.
The first involved a man about 40 who presented with a partially degloved penis. Through his embarrassment he told me that his wife was away at her sister's and he had "felt the need for an organism", so he placed his member in the nozzle of the vacuum cleaner (where the attachments should fit), switched it on and lost penile skin before he could switch it off.
Classmates may remember that around then there was a TV commercial for a vacuum cleaner which "beats as it sweeps as it cleans".
David Essenhigh, the consultant, wondered aloud if it had been one of those.
The second involved a man of 19 who, for reasons clear only to him, took a can of cavity wall filler foam, inserted the nozzle into his urethral meatus and pressed the button. The foam quickly set, presumably because his body temperature was much higher than that on a building site, making a perfect cast of his entire urethra. It would have been an excellent teaching aid had I not had to remove it piecemeal through multiple urethrotomies, as well as a suprapubic incision to remove some which had made its way to his bladder.

The last was tragic. A man in his late twenties was admitted from Walkergate Hospital where he was being treated for TB. On the morning "obs." round a nurse found him pale and shocked. She pulled back the bedclothes to find the bed half full of blood and his severed penis lying between his thighs.

His girlfriend, embarrassingly a nursing officer in NGH, had visited the previous evening and told him she did not wish to see him again. He had become acutely disturbed, decided that if the relationship was over, he would no longer need his penis, taken a razor blade and severed the redundant member.

Although he showed no other symptoms, I have assumed this was some transient acute schizoid episode precipitated by the distress.

He had arrived in the ambulance accompanied by a Tupperware box containing his penis on ice, but surgical techniques then did not allow re-attachment with the vascular and neurological anastomoses which would be needed, so the penis had to be discarded and the defect simply closed by bringing up the scrotal skin. It occurred to me later that leaving a man in his twenties with testes, but no penis was pretty cruel.

If ethics and the law had allowed, it might have been kinder to remove his testes and with them the urge to do something which he would never be able to do again. I do not know what became of him after I left Newcastle, but by ten years later he could have been treated by construction of a fat-filled skin tube and insertion of an inflatable prosthesis: a very poor substitute but (only just) better than nothing.

My first domiciliary visit

Many of the year will remember the Domiciliary Visit, whereby a consultant could be asked by a GP to visit a patient at home. I believe they were originally intended for those who could not travel for an outpatient consultation.

When properly done they involved the GP and consultant meeting at the patient's home, the consultant being introduced to the patient, doing the consultation, then withdrawing to discuss the problem with the GP who then interpreted the great man's opinion for the patient. By the time I started consultant practice (1977) most of this had been abandoned. The system was widely used as a means of jumping the outpatient queue and getting the patient into hospital quicker; and the GP was almost never there.

Consultants did not object as it attracted a generous fee and in Tayside it often meant a nice run into spectacular scenery (my farthest patient lived near Kinloch Rannoch, 85 miles by road from my base).

One of my general surgical colleagues always took a particular member of nursing staff with him on rural visits if the patient were female "in case I need a chaperone". Even allowing for the distances, some of his visits took, in the words of one of her (probably jealous) Dundonian colleagues, "an awfie lang time: he must be slow at the driving, ye ken".

Shortly after I took up my consultant post my Monday morning mail contained a small envelope bearing a second-class stamp and posted five days earlier. Inside was the visiting card of one of the city's less progressive GPs. On the back was a man's name, followed by the name of a care home run by Catholic nuns, and "? Retention of urine. Please do a DV and advise". Thinking that retention of urine might be more urgent than the mode of request suggested, I decided to go at once. Lacking a decent suit, I donned a new white coat, put a glove, KY Jelly and a catheter pack in my new briefcase and set off from Dundee Royal infirmary.

I digress here to give background to the end of this tale. Ninewells Hospital had opened three years earlier, and the major specialities had moved into it, but the old Royal Infirmary remained open and housed Urology and some other specialities. (At my interview in 1976 I was told that the Infirmary would close in 1980, when we would move to Ninewells.

In true NHS fashion that happened in 1998). Until my arrival the Dundee hospitals were, by a good few years, the last teaching hospitals in Britain not to have a trained and accredited urological surgeon. The general surgeons did the urology, sometimes with interesting results. After my arrival I was made forcefully aware that a conservative minority of them were unconvinced of the need for a specialist. Between urology at the Infirmary and some general surgeons at Ninewells there was tension, occasionally verging on open hostility.

I arrived at the care home, an ancient building which looked like the set of a gothic horror film, pulled on an iron bellpull and had the huge door creakily opened by a nun.

Before I could speak, she said "Come in, I'll get Mother Superior". I stood in a gloomy entrance hall lit by a shaft of sunlight coming from a high cupola, resplendent in new white coat and holding my Samsonite briefcase. There was a rustle of clothing and an imposing figure in full habit came along a corridor.

On seeing me she clapped her hands together and said in a broad Irish accent "Ah! 'tis the Rentokil man - God bless you for coming so soon!" Standing on my newly appointed dignity I pointed out that I was a Consultant Urological Surgeon come to see Mr X. Her response added a second insult: "You are too late; they took him to Ninewells in an ambulance an hour ago". At least she did not ask me to stay and deal with the cockroaches.

A memorable domiciliary visit.

This was the only properly conducted domiciliary visit in my 28 years in consultant practice. I was telephoned by a GP in Kirriemuir, a market town 20 miles away. The Kirriemuir practice was very highly regarded by my colleagues in all specialities.

The GP had been consulted by a 78-year old man, widowed a few years earlier and complaining of tiredness. In those days people in rural Angus troubled their doctors only when properly unwell: this man's Hb was 6g/dl, with a normochromic, normocytic pattern, and a creatinine eight times the upper limit.

The GP did a rectal examination and found an extensive stage 4 prostatic cancer which he assumed was occluding the ureters and causing the renal failure.

He knew that this was incurable, but that an orchidectomy, the treatment at the time, could give worthwhile remission (median 18 months) but his patient refused to go to hospital despite being told the prognosis if he did not. Would I see him at home and try to persuade him?

At 6pm I met the GP at his surgery and was driven to his patient's house on a council estate. As we went up the front garden path, I noticed the garden was entirely given over to vegetables, in immaculate neat rows with not a weed in sight. The door was opened by a ghastly pale, frail elderly man.

The GP said "Mr McPherson, this is the specialist from Dundee that I said I wanted you to see". The story would lose something if I did not report what happened next, verbatim.

The patient said in a gentle and matter-of-fact way "Aye, well I have just put my tea on the table so if you could fuck off and come back in an hour that would be braw" and closed the door.
The GP was profusely apologetic. I was amused and suggested we passed the hour in The Strathmore Arms. We returned an hour later and were invited in as if there had been no previous contact. I confirmed the GP's findings, and the patient confirmed his absolute refusal to be admitted. I left, having promised to admit him at once if he changed his mind.
Five days later the GP telephoned to say his patient had died, but not before telling him that the refusal of admission was due to his vegetable garden. It was his pride and joy and only source of pleasure. He knew that if he went into hospital the local youths would have his garden stripped bare before the ambulance was out of town. I realised that I had been given something rare for surgeons but common for GPs: an insight into someone's life beyond their illness.
After more experience, having had elderly patients tell me that each night they prayed that they would not wake the next morning, it occurred to me that there might be another explanation. He was a tired widower who had had enough of life and wanted to put down the burden: perhaps the vegetables were an acceptable excuse.

A trip on a ship

After house jobs I became a demonstrator in anatomy, the first rung on the surgical ladder. To supplement my income I did, like several of us, GP surgeries.
Some of these (at three guineas for a 35-patient evening surgery, five guineas for a Saturday morning) were at a practice in Wallsend where one partner was also MO to the Swan Hunter shipyard. He offered me the chance to do a five-day trip on a newly-built ship undergoing sea trials. Five days of work would bring the equivalent of a month's salary.
I reported at the shipyard early one afternoon and was taken on board by a director of Swan Hunter. It was clear the ship was run very much on the principle of "Officers" and "Other ranks". The "officers" were SH directors, the future captain and chief engineer of the ship (a refrigerated transport for Fyffe's bananas), directors of Fyffe's and myself. For the directors this was a jolly; no work and five days of eating and especially drinking.

We were to be looked after by a chef and three stewards, who were not SH employees. One director had a contact who was a dining-car steward at British Rail. When such a trip was planned the BR steward contacted three colleagues and on the day before the trip they all called in sick and set off for Wallsend.

My first contact with the stewards was later that first afternoon. I went on deck to find three of them gathered by the rail. They were outrageously flamboyant effeminate homosexuals who referred to each other as “she” and wore make-up. I had never come across anything like this in my 25 years.

In those days anyone who was homosexual (“gay” had not then been appropriated) kept it quiet if they did not wish to be beaten up in the street. Perhaps these folks were only able to be themselves in this environment, and I suspect they were also camping it up for the benefit of the “officers”.

They were on deck because one of their number, the chef, had missed the boat’s departure and was being brought out in a cutter (by this time we were a mile off Whitley Bay). A rope ladder was put over the side. There was a swell on, and the cutter was rising and falling by several feet, so there was much squealing and protesting by the chef about the difficulty of getting onto the ladder. One steward turned to a director and said in a voice that Larry Grayson would have envied “If that girl gets upset, there will be no food served on this boat tonight, I can tell you”, but all went well eventually, and I went to my cabin having been exposed to something totally new to me.

The stewards and chef looked after us very well, and the food was magnificent. I shall return to them at the end of this tale.

My other memory is of the prodigious alcohol consumption, in which I was, as one of the “officers”, expected to participate. I had been told to report to the wardroom at 6.30 for drinks before dinner. Everyone was drinking huge measures of gin, to which some added a splash of tonic.

The captain took his neat. I had never tasted gin, finding the smell of it unpleasant, but not wishing to let the side down I accepted some and found it pleasant with the addition of about five times as much tonic as the others were using.

As soon as a glass neared empty a steward refilled it. I quickly developed a practice, which had to be continued for the rest of the trip, of raising the glass to my lips and opening them but drinking only a tiny sip. Dinner was accompanied by generous glasses of wine and followed by brandy, again in large measure. Despite my prophylactic manoeuvres I returned to my cabin fervently hoping that my professional services would not be needed. In fact, I had nothing whatever to do in the whole trip.

At noon on the first full day a steward, who had the hotel chambermaid's knack of knocking on a door and simultaneously opening it, told me that "Drinks before lunch Sir" would be in the wardroom at 12.30. The ethanolic sequence of the previous evening was repeated, as it was at each subsequent lunch and dinner. After lunch I returned to my cabin and an hour later a steward appeared with "Your afternoon beer, Sir" and handed over four bottles of Newcastle Exhibition Ale and an opener.

I was concerned: was I really expected to drink a bottle of beer between two very alcoholic meals, each afternoon for the remaining four days? Of course not: the four bottles were just for that day; four more appeared each afternoon. Not one was opened. I felt badly about this alcohol consumption by the "officers", because below decks were over a hundred men working hard in unpleasant, hot conditions testing engines etc. and if any of them was found to have consumed, or be in possession of, alcohol they were sent ashore in disgrace. The directors did nothing but drank enough to float the ship. The demise of ship-building on the Tyne was blamed on a mixture of cheaper foreign competition and restrictive Trades Union practices, but I have often wondered if the attitudes and state of those in charge of the companies was at least a factor.

On the last day we were due to dock after lunch. Just after breakfast I was approached by two burly riggers:" Got any Plaster of Paris doc?".

My makeshift sick bay did have a large box of those dry bandages impregnated with gypsum which were soaked in water to make a plaster cast. My inquiry as to what they wanted it for was met with "Make sure you stay to the end of lunch". I was not going to need it by then so I said they could take some. They took the box.

At the end of lunch, a director rose to say words of thanks to the stewards. As he did so a rigger entered with the cardboard box which had contained the plaster bandages. From it he took an erect phallus, well over two feet long, complete with testes, all skilfully made from Plaster of Paris. It was very lifelike apart from its colour (and size). It was presented to the chef, who accepted it with squeals of delight against a background of ribald comments from the others about what he would be doing when he got it home.
So, the "officers", at least, disembarked happy and entertained. The directors divided up the left-over alcohol. Despite the gargantuan consumption there was enough for each to take home what to me seemed a six-month supply. I left happy to have not had some horrific accident to deal with and anticipating my generous cheque, having had my eyes opened to an aspect of human behaviour hitherto unknown to me – and with a taste for gin.

An incident recalled – or not.
This tale is not from my clinical career; it happened well into retirement, but the best stories are told against oneself, so here goes. I am still a member of the BMA and read the BMJ, though the portion read diminishes almost weekly. My subscription is paid by direct debit in August. Five years ago, I realised in October that I had not had a BMJ for some weeks. I contacted BMA membership who, after some keyboard tapping, told me that because of a problem at their bank my direct debit had not been collected and because of this my membership had lapsed. I explained in a "full and frank" manner that I could understand one error, but to discontinue my membership rather than contacting me to sort it out, was something I found difficult to accept.
They explained that this was all done automatically by computer, and I brusquely pointed out that they had confirmed that "to err is human, but to really foul things up you need a computer". (As this tale shows, memory is fallible, so "foul" may not have been the word I used.) I got an apology and a promise to reinstate my membership backdated to August.
Two years ago, in October, I again realised that I had not had a BMJ for some weeks. I assumed there had been a repeat of the previous episode and contacted BMA membership, having mentally prepared the dressing-down which they richly deserved.

After more keyboard tapping, I was put on hold and a few minutes later an obviously more senior voice came on.
"I understand that you are concerned that you no longer receive the BMJ".
"I certainly am, and not for the first time".
"I shall read an email we had from you at 10.37 on 21st July: you wrote "I am appalled that the BMA is supporting junior doctors in taking industrial action in response to proposed changes to their way of working. Industrial action is never appropriate in the NHS, especially by doctors. I no longer wish to be a member of an organisation which acts in this way. I resign with immediate effect and have cancelled my direct debit".
I have to admit that he was at least halfway through before I remembered sending the email. Until then I had total absence of recall of something which I had felt strongly about all of three months earlier.
I made a humble apology to which he replied, "Don't worry doctor, it happens all the time": a considerate but obviously untrue response, and at least he did not add "... when we are dealing with senile buggers such as yourself". My membership was again reinstated.
I put down the phone reflecting that, approaching 75, I had left it rather late to correct my lifelong fault of jumping to paranoid conclusions (well, at least I have insight). It later occurred to me that this total absence of recall might be the first step down the slippery slope which we dread. I was going to say "Thankfully there have been no other instances" but how do I know there are not more out there, waiting to come to light? But I can say I *know* of no other instances - if I ignore the perpetually missing mobile phone and car keys.

A few random quickies.
In urology at NGH we checked patients' post vasectomy semen samples ourselves by direct microscopy in the clinic. One patient brought a pot (full) of what was obviously urine. I explained to him, in the most basic terms I could summon, what we actually needed. I guarantee this to be true: next week he brought a pot (full) of......faeces. A further chat by a Geordie male nurse made it " third time lucky".

Talking of providing samples, a recently circulated WhatsApp funny was from a supposed sperm donor: "I went to donate, and the nurse said, " Would you like to ejaculate in the cup?". I said," Well I am pretty good, but I don't think I am ready for a competition just yet". It would be improper to give " interesting" patients' names if they were still alive, but neither of these can be. A contact in blood transfusion said he had just signed a letter to a donor from Newcastle's Jewish community, saying that he had reached the age when donations were no longer accepted: a Mr Hyman Bender. I relayed this to David Essenhigh when I was his SR in 1973. He countered with the fact that in his student days he had clerked a Mr Janus, whose parents had thoughtfully named him Hugh.

In the late 70s a local GP had a letter in the BMJ explaining why KY jelly was so-called, at least in Scotland. It suggested that when the old ladies went into the chemists to buy it, they waited until the shop was empty and approached the assistant with "Er... Ken Yon jelly? .... The BMJ would not publish that now.

For some years in the 80's I was visiting professor of urology at Louisiana State University Medical School in Shreveport, up near the Arkansas border: an interesting experience in time travel. The local urologists had two quips which they used on any excuse. Jimmy Carter had recently been President. Their consensus opinion was that "Whoever circumcised him threw away the wrong bit". The other was about the Mexican who, after his prostatectomy, had the inevitable retrograde ejaculation. "They called him Dry Martinez".

Ivan Carrington

Early times.

I was on a three-year trial period in a GP practice in Brighton in the mid to late 70's and they were the Police Surgeons to East Sussex constabulary for Brighton & Hove. My mistake was thinking that any call outs would be at chucking out time in the pubs as most of the work was taking bloods after a positive breathalyser but in fact it usually was more like 3 AM.

Brighton is a serious place for crime. One Sunday on call over lunch the phone rings from the police saying I am required to confirm a death and is it suspicious or not. I say can I finish my lunch and I will be along after that? NO, get here Now. Unfriendly type but OK will do. Find the road on my A-Z, back of the Town Hall Hove. Get there, police tape and flashing lights from police cars fill the road and looking like a police drama. Wind window down,

"I am the police surgeon" I say.

"Yes, this way."

As we go through the back entrance to the town hall, I cannot help noticing that everyone has a handkerchief over their mouth.

(By the way we were in the height of summer and it was hot.)

It wasn't that difficult to confirm death of the Mayor of Hove but rolling him over to look at his back in case I missed a knife or bullet wound was strange, as the skin or rather the S\C tissue was a bit liquid. I have never seen so many blue bottles, they were everywhere! It was only when I got out into the fresh air did I realise how I was soaked in sweat and almost threw up. Poor devil everyone thought he had gone on holiday, but he had died I hope peacefully, in his bed.

On finishing my registration year and now a fully trained proper doctor I had a few months to fill-in before heading to Glasgow to be an Anatomy Demonstrator. Seems crazy looking back to go and forget quite a bit of acute medicine. Somehow through word of mouth I was taken on as a GP locum in South Shields, with two weeks for one partner and two weeks for the other. I don't think I was much use.

I was put up in the working partner's house in great luxury and fed and watered.

In my second fortnight I stayed with the senior partner and always remember his dining room where we spent quite a bit of time as it was paneled in the best mahogany taken from ships that were being broken in the yards on the Tyne.

He lived and worked his life in South Shields so had the contacts and was a pillar of local society. I did my rounds in a self-constructed Ford Special and it was very rough, but it did work. The instrument binnacle was from a Jag, but the speedo wasn't connected as the gearing was all different and the cable end going from a Jaguar instrument to a Ford gearbox wouldn't fit.

One day said senior partner asked if I could give him a lift somewhere local so he lowered his large frame into the passenger's side where at that stage of construction I had recently fitted a seat which was OK. He was a practical man and very observant as driving through town he noticed my speedo wasn't working so how did I know I was observing the speed limit? Hopefully quick as a flash I pointed out that doing the maths from the electronic rev counter knowing the gearing in 4th gear I would know what speed the car was going. He just nodded. Incidentally he was the senior magistrate. I couldn't look him in the eye for a day or two afterwards.

In 1980 I was appointed as a single-handed GP to a lovely practice on the edge of the Cotswold's and I finished nearly 30 years later with a partner and a salaried. It was hard work being on 24/7 and learning about the family dynamics of the locals which was fascinating. Early on at some function in one of the villages to meet the "new doctor" I was hugged by a middle-aged lady from one of the local families who seem to make up a significant part of the village population. Populations were still fairly stable then.

"Oh, doctor aren't you lovely, I am sure I can help you with your work just don't hesitate to ask" or something along those lines.

I also met someone with the same family name who I think was a cousin. My receptionist later told me that these two ladies loathe one another so just be careful what I say. Anyhow, that same evening I was informed that the lady giving out the warm hugs and who was a bit cracked was in fact the village "Midwife", untrained but probably very necessary in local communities where there was no state midwife or doctor. She passed away only a few weeks ago.

How times have changed.

Khurshed Dastur

My time with Freddie Mercury

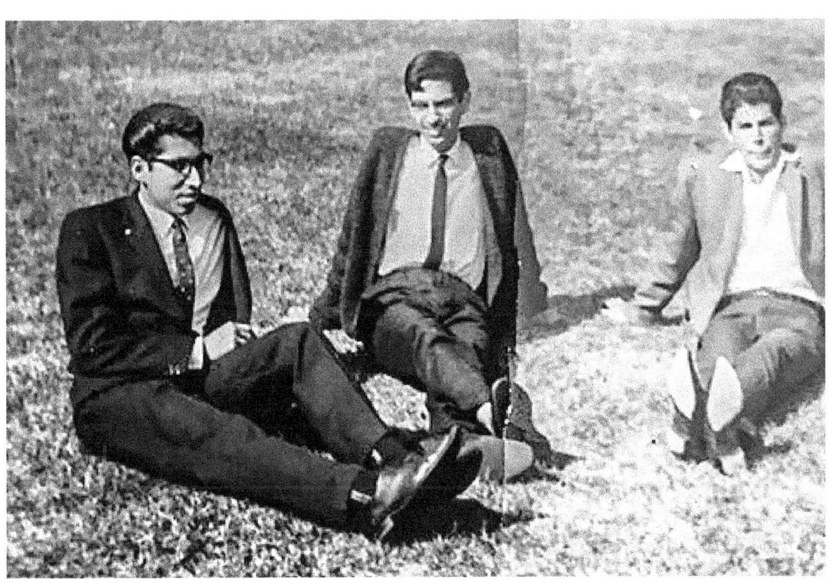

1964 picture of myself (on the left) with Freddie Mercury (on the right with his buck teeth).

At that time Freddie had just arrived in England and was studying Graphic Designing at the Ealing College of Arts in London. We were both born in Zanzibar a couple of houses from each other and had grown up together.
He was sent to a boarding school in India, and I met him again in London in 1964 when I was a second year medical student in Newcastle.
He asked my friend Percy (sitting in the middle and also from Zanzibar) if he could join his band and Percy said,
"Freddie forget it you have no talent"!!
History proved different but they remained friends till Freddie passed many years later.

God moves in mysterious ways.

As it was very cold in my flat in Chester Crescent in Jesmond during the winter months, I used to study till late at night in the RVI in the cafeteria below Lecture Theatre One. A few of us in similar circumstances poured over the books there and I still remember Lawrence Warbara and I grilling each other. One wintry night at about eleven o clock I left the RVI and started walking to my flat. I decided to take a short cut to go towards the Town Hall by crossing the bus stands in Hay Market. I stepped down not realising a bus was coming into park and was flung forward and hit the railings and fell to the ground. The wheel of the double decker stopped about six inches from my chest. The bus driver shouted," wait I am going to back out". He had gone over my brief case in my outstretched hand and thinking it was me backed over it again. When he stepped out of the bus, he was paler than me and asked me if I was ok. My glasses had gone flying and on getting up fell to the ground again. But I got a hold of myself and stood up again.

A policeman standing near the theatre on the other side of the street saw what had happened and came running over and asked me if I was ok and told me to go get myself checked out in the emergency room in the RVI.

So, I walked back to the hospital on that slightly snowy night cursing the cop for not driving me. In the emergency room the son of one of our famous ENT consultants examined my painful right wrist and glibly told me nothing was wrong and to go home.

So again, I walked back to my flat. As I could not sleep from the pain, I went back to the emergency room next morning and an x ray revealed a right radial styloid fracture. A plaster cast was immediately applied from the base of the thumb to just above the elbow.

It was hell for a month as I am right handed. Luckily the late Harry Bell and some others who sat next to me took notes for me as I could not write. On that wintry night I think God spared me and said my time was not up and made that double decker bus wheel just stop short and gave me a second life as I think he wanted me to be a physician!!

An American career.

Having graduated in 1968 and following a house job at the RVI under Professor Smart and Taffy Jones I decided to go to America for further training. Because of my three-month externship in the States in our fourth year at the Morrisania city hospital which was part of Montefiore Hospital in New York I was told by the chief on my last day that if I wanted there was a job waiting for me upon graduation. However, because the Vietnam war was going on, I decided to go to Edmonton Canada till the war was over.

In the Royal Alexandra hospital there one day I was assigned as an intern to the medical ICU. One day I was tending to an extremely sick individual and realised that he would soon be breathing his last, so I summoned the Chaplain to come to the ICU to give him the Last Rights.

Having done that, I was unfortunately called to assist a cardiac arrest a few beds down. While performing CPR I saw from the corner of my eye the Chaplain enter the ICU. However, I noticed immediately that he had stopped at the wrong bed and was administering the last rights to the wrong patient. Unable to leave the patient I was administering the CPR to I asked the nurse assisting me to pull him away from the bed where he was administering the last rights before the patient or the visiting family would realise what was going on! I believe nowadays it is no longer called the last rights but the sacrament of the sick.

After two years in Canada, I went to Pittsburgh in the States and changed to radiology and became a neuroradiologist after learning how to do studies like angiograms, pneumoencephalograms and myelograms. I got puked upon doing many a pneumoencephalogram. It was the most barbaric study ever invented as we had to summersault and reverse summersault the poor patient strapped down in his chair after we had injected air in his lumbar spine. Needless to say, the patient never came back for a repeat study. The advent of the CAT scanner ended the era of pneumo-encephalograms for the patient and the radiologist and what a relief!!

My speeding record in Pittsburgh was dismal as I had to be in the hospital in half an hour for stroke or trauma call. One day my sister in law Lilly Dastur was stopped for speeding not too far from my house.

The policeman said to Lilly just a minute and went to his patrol car to check her driving record on the computer. He came back and surprisingly asked her "are you related to Dr Dastur?" She with a straight face denied she knew me. She escaped with just a warning!
I fell asleep twice in 40 years driving to and from work. One day surprisingly going to the hospital in the morning I rammed a pickup truck in front of me at a fairly low speed as it was a busy street and raining cats and dogs. I was petrified as I expected a huge brawl. To my surprise a well-suited gentleman got out of the pickup truck and came running towards my car. I was prepared for the worst but thanks to the rain and the man realising there was no significant damage to his truck he turned round yelling at me and got back into his pickup truck and drove away. A close encounter!
I used to have a personalised licence plate on my BMW. NUROMRI it read. Again, one day going home I dozed off and rear ended an old lady's car. She turned into the nearby street and got out of the car. Seeing my licence plate, she started asking me if I was ok and if I was a neurosurgeon!! I said no just a neuroradiologist and apologised even though there was no damage to her car as we were doing a couple of miles an hour as it was peak traffic time. To my surprise she thanked me for stopping. That was the awe and respect we commanded!
My telling a magistrate I was dragged in front of once that I have treated many a cop and even the sheriff of the county infuriated him so much that he got out of his chair demanding what that had to do with the proceedings. I said I had paid the fine and was looking for a waiver of points and he shouted even if it was in his power to do so he would not. I left the courthouse dejected but a few months later I was glad to read in the local paper that he was thrown off the bench because of drunkenness.
God protects us in mysterious ways!
About three years into my first job, I became chief of neuroradiology as my boss suddenly decided to take another appointment outside of Pittsburgh. As a neuroradiologist I was asked to perform an angiogram on a patient with a residual frontal lobe benign meningioma.
I found out the patient had been operated previously at an outside hospital by a very prominent neurosurgeon and my neuroradiology predecessor had also done a postoperative angiogram on this individual.

My neurosurgeon then had reoperated on this patient again with only partial success.
One day sometime later this patient, who I was convinced had become frontal lobish from the surgeries, walked into a local church and told the pastor he was going to kill the first neurosurgeon who had operated on him. The pastor informed the neurosurgeon who immediately left town.
Then after a few days the patient started calling my department and asking first for my predecessor and then me. I told my secretary not to take his calls. On making further enquiries I found out he had been calling my neurosurgeon's office as well and the office of other medical and neurology consultants who had been involved in his care. I found out all these doctors had bought guns. Never having owned or fired a gun I decided it would not be wise for me to do so. I told my wife 'do not open the door if anybody appears at the front door'.
Later one day I talked to the chief of Neurosurgery. I could not believe when he said to me that all the detectives in the city knew about this chap and what he was doing but unless he put a hand on one of us nothing could be done. I said thanks a lot!!
A couple of years later my Interventional Radiology colleague, a great angiographer but very timid suddenly walked into my office and asked me to talk to his patient whom he had just angiogramed for leg ischemia and was yelling obscenities at him. I first looked at the chart and immediately realised that it was the same patient. Unfortunately, the patient had developed a huge hematoma in the groin due to inadequate compression of the femoral artery post angiogram. We consulted with the chief of Vascular Surgery who decided to admit the patient overnight. The hospital security was immediately notified as well.
I had developed the nasty habit of reading every day the obituary column in the local newspaper. One fine day a couple of years later I read the patient's name in this column. The neurosurgical office staff confirmed it was the dreaded man.
We were all relieved and the drinks flowed freely at the local bar that evening.

John Davies

Early Days

After graduation, I headed to York for my pre-registration house posts at the City Hospital. After six years in Medical School this was what it was all about. It is hard to explain to non-medicals the feeling of pride of wandering the empty hospital corridors at night knowing that you are Doctor Davies, House Physician/Surgeon, and you are in charge, albeit with your Registrar at the end of the telephone. It doesn't take long for the gloss to wear off after a few sleepless nights. In York, there was no dedicated Paediatric ward, so children were housed in an annexe adjoining the general ward and I had to cover for them at night. To this day, I have never forgotten two teenagers with terminal illnesses who spent their last few weeks of life on the ward. I developed a rapport talking with them during quiet periods on duty and, over 50 years later, I can still see their faces and remember their quiet acceptance of their fate.

One of the duties of the House Officer was to take the calls from GPs requesting hospital admission for their patients and I sometimes look back in shame at my attempts as a newly qualified doctor to persuade, out of hours, someone with far more experience than myself, that an admission could possibly wait until morning. Usually there was little doubt that it would not wait.

Six months as Surgical House Officer introduced me to some of the more unusual emergencies that had not been covered in the Medical School curriculum. The York City Hospital housed General Surgery and Medicine, which included most of the sub specialities that now have their own dedicated teams and Consultancies. The Consultants were generalists with special interests. Casualty (Not A&E in those days) was in York General Hospital, the older of the two establishments and situated around a mile down the road. If the Casualty Officer wished to admit a patient, I had to get in my car and go and take a look. During my six months in post, there were three particular instances that "stand out" and they all show the ingenious lengths to which some men will go in order to achieve sexual gratification and the lack of foresight into the consequences.

The insertion into the urethra of a ball point pen did not pose too many problems of retrieval but a bead-ended hat pin had to be removed by the trans-vesical route.

The worst however was the vacuum cleaner injury, which I am told is not unusual. Patients can come up with ingenious explanations when they come to grief. In this case the victim explained that he was up in the bedroom mending the vacuum cleaner and accidentally dropped a live lead and electrocuted his penis. The patient was transferred to the City Hospital where he was prepared for repair under GA. Deep down, I know that it is wrong to derive humour from the afflictions of one's patients but over the course of my career it has sometimes been a very useful coping mechanism at times of adversity. In this case, when he was on the table and his mutilated member protruded from the green surgical towels, the likeness to the Loch Ness Monster was striking. I think we spent as much time photographing it as we did in removing all the pieces of chrome from his wounds and repairing the damage.

It was around this time that I first became aware of the ignorance of NHS Management of the importance of supporting the good will of the staff, without which the Health Service could not survive. There was an occasion when the air conditioning in the theatre was not working but we soldiered on in difficult conditions and at a break between patients, the Consultant sent down to one of the wards to acquire a bottle of orange juice with which to rehydrate the team. At the end of the month a bill for this arrived, addressed to "The Theatre Staff". The said Consultant tore it up muttering under his breath that he would make an issue of it at the next appropriate opportunity. Another time I found myself around 2 am, having had no break since the previous lunchtime. A routine afternoon list had gone on till the evening, following which the Registrar and I dealt with a few emergencies that had come in during the day. I then had to clerk some of the new admissions before turning in for the day. As I was finishing, I took a call from a GP on the periphery of our catchment area and had to accept an admission in the knowledge that it would take around two hours for my patient to arrive. There was no point in going to bed, so I sent a message to the kitchen asking if there were any meals left over from the night staff's lunch break. They were happy to oblige but at the end of the month the cost of the meal was deducted from my pay cheque.

It seemed that it was all right for me to soldier on for well over a normal working day, but any extra sustenance required was at my own expense.

I had become used to the disturbed nights which would become a feature of the rest of my career, but nothing prepared me for my next job in Obstetrics, the busiest time of my entire career during which I reckoned I averaged around four hours sleep a night, one night in two. The main reason was the requirement for all episiotomies and lacerations to be sutured by a doctor. For some reason, even the most experienced midwife was not to be entrusted with this task. I got to the stage where I asked the staff not to engage me in conversation, in the hope that I could complete the repair without fully waking up. A few well practiced words of support and explanation to the patient came automatically. The experience, however, was invaluable for a future in General Practice. I had planned to follow up this post with six months in anaesthetics. In York there was a well-trodden path for future GPs of Medicine, Surgery, Obstetrics and Anaesthetics, because providing gassing services to local Dentists was quite a lucrative side-line. One lunchtime however I was approached at a postgraduate meeting by a local GP with the opening "Are you the Doctor Davies we have heard so much about?" Flattery will only go so far but the promise of a considerable increase in income if I filled a vacancy in his practice in Selby, was too much to turn down. I therefore skipped the Anaesthetics and took my first tentative steps in the career that I would pursue for the rest of my working life.

An Introduction to Family Medicine.

In those days there was no requirement to do any form of vocational training, so I turned up on day one at the surgery situated in the house of the retired Senior Partner, whose shoes I was expected to fill, albeit as a mere "Assistant With View". I was given a prescription pad and told to get on with it. Fortunately, there was nothing on the morning list too challenging although when a mother came in dragging a small child with the opening remark "Ee's got Gerbils doctor", I struggled for a while. Obviously, I had heard of Measles and Chicken pox but not Gerbils. My blushes were spared when she followed up with "and one of 'ems bitten 'im!".

I was relieved to have survived my first couple of hours in Practice without mishap and headed to the lounge only to find that the other partners had long since finished, had their coffees and gone out on their rounds leaving me a list of patients requiring home visits.

I worked my way round these with the help of a map of the area and went home for lunch.

That afternoon I returned to the surgery to find that two of my morning visits had immediately asked for a follow up by "a proper doctor". The solution was right in front of my nose. I would try to make myself look older by growing a moustache.
Days were long as the Practice held three unstaffed branch surgeries in neighbouring villages with sessions held at the beginning and end of the day. The doctors dispensed to these patients but there were no records held on the premises so repeat prescriptions were quite challenging. Large cardboard "hat boxes" contained pills such as Aspirin, Paracetamol, Thyroxine, Digoxin and Dig. Fol., which looked as if it was made of crushed foxglove leaves and probably was. The patient would bring a small pill box which was scooped into the larger box to replenish their supply having deduced by questioning what was the most likely medication. Likewise, liquid medications were dispensed from large Winchester bottles containing various ancient stomach mixtures or opiate-containing bronchial elixirs. If the patient's bottle had not been washed out, an educated guess could be made as to its contents by viewing and sniffing or tasting the dregs. If it was clean, the patient could be invited to sniff from the Winchester to help with identification.
My stay at Selby lasted only nine months, ending by mutual agreement. It is said that in General Practice, you need to take more care in choosing your future partners than you do your spouse, and I did not feel that I wanted to spend the rest of my career working with these fellows. It was time to view the situations vacant pages of the BMJ. I could never understand the reluctance in these advertisements to give the exact location so "Pleasant North East Coastal Practice" resulted in me heading for interview to Redcar for a post in a three-man practice. I was pleased to be offered the position.

A New Start by the Seaside

The town at the time was indeed pleasant, despite being in the shadow of the giant steel works and, compared to my experience in Selby, everyone was friendly.
We arrived at the beginning of December and within days were invited to the Christmas dinner dances of the Rugby Club, Swimming Club, Cricket Club, the Catenians (a sort of Catholic Rotary Club) and the Stead Hospital, a small local hospital endowed by a local benefactor of that name.

The hospital dance was quite amusing as Matron was married to the owner of one of the many Italian ice cream establishments in the town and he had invited a number of his fellow traders with the result that the top table looked like a scene from "The Godfather". In my attempts to modify my boyish good looks and make myself look a little older, I grew a beard and in fact I have had one on and off for most of my adult life. On one such transitional occasion, I was making a return visit to a patient after a week during which I had shaved one off, only to be greeted by the gruff comment "Oh God, not another new doctor. I hope you are better than the last one, the one with the beard. He was rubbish!" In those days home visits were commonplace and one's paperback-sized visiting diary could be full of follow-ups even before the day's new requests were added. I am reminded of one such a revisit to a woman with a bad back who I had advised the week before to stay in bed (remember those days?). As was usual, after a cursory knock I let myself in and climbing the stairs to her bedroom, I heard a shout from the ground floor. "I'm down here you silly bugger!" Descending the stairs and entering the back room I was greeted by a surprised patient. "I'm so sorry Doctor, I thought you were the milkman."

My senior partner in Redcar was an interesting character. As a young outspoken Austrian in the early 1940s with strong anti-Nazi views, he had been urged by his family to leave the country for his own safety. He arrived in the UK and joined the Army Medical Corps. His superiors urged him to change his name from Franz Mandel and called him instead Frank Morley, lest his fellow soldiers thought he was German. That must have been quite a leap of faith because even 30 years later, he couldn't have looked more Germanic had he taken to wearing lederhosen.

After the war he had entered Medical School and on graduation obtained a position of "Assistant With View" in a two-man practice in the Redcar satellite of Dormanstown.

It would appear that the Senior Partner was fairly obviously suffering from mental illness and alcoholism, enough to have him struck off the Medical Register, but as was the norm in those days his colleagues turned a blind eye. Frank was one in a long line of assistants who, when the time came for consideration of partnership, were accused of some major misdemeanour, such as raping their employer's wife, and were sent packing with no money.

When his time came, Frank was approached by a deputation of patients asking him to set up in practice in opposition, with the incentive of rent-free premises for a surgery. He did this and very quickly acquired a sizeable list of patients deserting the old practice. Thirty years later he was still loved by his patients even when they were being forcibly admonished for failing to follow his advice. I was very fond of Frank who, with two daughters, I believe looked upon me as the son he never had. The feeling became mutual when, two years after joining the practice, my own father died suddenly on holiday in Austria. It was therefore with considerable mixed feelings when after eight years in Redcar, I decided to move on.
Although by now, along with all the local practices, we had moved into a purpose-built Health Centre in the centre of Redcar, a sizeable proportion of our patients lived in Dormanstown. Originally a village of superior housing built for workers in the neighbouring steel works of Dorman Long, it had latterly been used to rehouse families from the slum clearances on the edge of Middlesbrough and the Police had asked that all the problem families be kept together so that they could be more easily monitored. When I was on call in the evening and out on visits, Val, my wife, would often be verbally abused on the telephone when I was not immediately available. That, along with some differences of opinion I was having with one of my other partners that resulted in me coming home at the end of the day and grumbling over the dinner table, was enough for Val to issue an ultimatum to do something about it or shut up. My son was about to move on to secondary school, so it seemed a good time to make the move. I had always had a yen to be in the countryside, so it was back to the ads in the BMJ.

A Move to the Country

To cut a long story short, "Pleasant Village on The Edge of The North York Moors" turned out to be Great Ayton, boyhood home of Captain James Cook, and I was pleased to become an "Assistant With View" there. From being a full partner in a large town practice to an assistant at a small rural practice resulted in a considerable drop in income but looking back I don't regret it one bit. Without a rota with a neighbouring practice, being on duty one night or weekend in three was quite a reality check but when home visits involved driving through some of the most attractive countryside, the slight loss of freedom was a price worth paying.

Having worked in the Practice for nearly 30 years, like most doctors, I remember many highs and lows, comedies and tragedies although for the purpose of this account, I would prefer to avoid the latter. Comedic situations abound and usually at the patient's expense, so I soon developed coping mechanisms to avoid showing my inward feelings. Taking out a handkerchief out under the pretense of blowing my nose, I could often conceal a chuckle and pulling my nasal hairs at the same time could restore a sense of decorum. There have been many such incidences too numerous to recount but two in particular spring to mind. The patient who arrived in surgery with a post vasectomy haematoma and on dropping his trousers revealed his "crown jewels" to be protected by a rabbit jelly mould was one such incident that required all my powers of self-control. Another was a consultation with a middle-aged man who had plucked up courage to see me regarding his recent impotence. "I don't know Doctor. It might be normal for my age, but I don't have a yardstick to measure it by".

Another incident concerned one of my partners. Being in a one-in-three rota had a considerable negative affect on one's social life but as call-outs were infrequent and, providing I remained sober I could attend social activities when on call. The occasion was my 50th birthday party and as there were several in attendance who did not know each other, I had given everyone a sticky label with their name on it. During the course of the evening, my partner, Brian, was called as an emergency to someone who had collapsed and died in an outside toilet. He had to climb in through the window to examine the deceased before manhandling him away from the door to enable it to be opened. After the patient was removed, Brian returned to the party. The following morning, during coffee break, there was a call from the Coroner's Officer for clarification of the patient's identity. On his arrival at the mortuary, he had a sticky label with "Brian" on it, obviously transferred during the events of the night before. Sad for the patient but light relief for the doctors.

Christmas in General Practice is a time of mixed feelings. Being on duty when everyone else is getting merry is quite sobering, literally, but it has its lighter moments.

Visiting the local cottage hospital and doing a ward round on Christmas Day puts your own "inconvenience" into perspective and on one occasion while there, I was interviewed by the local radio station who were doing a feature on people working on the day.

I am also reminded of an occurrence that brings a smile to my face whenever I recount it.

It was the week before Christmas, and I had been asked to visit the elderly mother of a local farmer. The weather had been bad for several days and I set off for the farm thankful that I had not just washed the car. The area around the farm was about to be engulfed by the urban spread of the nearby town and the mile-long track had been turned into a quagmire by construction vehicles. I arrived looking like a fugitive from the RAC rally.

I crossed a muddy courtyard to be greeted at the back door by the farmer's wife, who invited me inside. Peering through a snowstorm of feathers, I could just make out the Christmas production line. Everywhere I looked there were turkeys. To my left, piled almost to the ceiling, were the corpses of recently killed birds. To my right, three women were plucking, cleaning and gutting, skillfully preparing the oven-ready product that occupied every other available space in this large farmhouse kitchen. Amid profuse apologies for the mess, I was led through to the hallway. Walking sideways, I carefully eased past more stacks of soon-to-be Christmas dinners and up the stairs to my patient.

I examined the old lady, prescribed an antibiotic for her acute bronchitis and attempted to retrace my steps through the scene of poultry carnage to my car. At the door I was thanked for my trouble and was halfway across the yard when I was called back. "Doctor, would you like a tur......" My spirits immediately lifted. GPs are fairly easily pleased. A few words of appreciation from a satisfied patient can make up for a surgery full of moaners. At Christmas however it is not unknown for the thank-you to take a more tangible form. It is amazing the number of thoughts that can pass through one's mind in the few microseconds between two syllables of a word, but my flights of fancy were abruptly grounded as the farmer's wife finished her sentence. "......a turnip?" she said, "Freshly cut today."

Ah well. It is the thought that counts.

Looking back over my career I consider myself truly fortunate to have been a GP at a time when it was indeed Family Medicine. I was responsible for delivering babies, both in two different GP maternity units and at the patient's home. I performed all the infant welfare checks and vaccinations. I developed friendships with patients of all ages, on one occasion having a regular home visit to a 103-year-old lady interrupted by a call to attend at the birth of the newest patient of the practice. Sometimes I had emergency calls to patients who, despite my best efforts, died in front of me and I had to comfort the relatives. I had the privilege of looking after the terminally ill, both in their own homes and in nursing homes. I could go on, but you get the point. Nowadays many of these activities have been taken over by other team members such as Health Visitors, Practice Nurses and Paramedics and many would say it is for the better, relieving GPs to perform other important duties such as management, budgeting and commissioning. Having had an overdraft for most of my working life, why anyone would trust me with managing a large budget, beats me, and anyway, if I had been that way inclined, I would have chosen accountancy over medicine. Would I advise a grandchild to go into General Practice? I am not sure now.

David Fieldhouse

YEAR OF '68 TREATISE

On the basis and in the hope that many of those reading this book may have little knowledge of medical terminology and the meaning of many signs and symptoms with which medics are familiar, I aim to use as much plain English as practicable in the following anthology.

IN THE BEGINNING

I am immeasurably fortunate to say that I have yet to get up in the morning – which has all too frequently been after far too little sleep – not looking forward to the day ahead. This seems to be such a unusual state of affairs as to be a rare medical syndrome. Perhaps I developed an immunity to melancholia at the start of the day by virtue either of the good fortune of surviving a bicycle crash into the front of the lorry WKW 477 – concussion, fractured collar bone, fractured skull (occiput) – prior to the start of Medical School or the cheating of death at the hands of the a surgical Registrar in Downpatrick who clearly had not absorbed his pharmacological teaching sufficiently to know that an injection of 1 ml of 1:1000 adrenaline into my left lower eyelid as part of his misunderstanding of the local anaesthetic required for the excision of my umpteenth chalazion (cyst in the eyelid), could have been fatal to me. It is a fact that all your life passes before you as you lay, dying, on the operating table and also that you forget it pretty quickly when you realise that you have survived it, fifteen minutes later, and the operation ensues with the prospect of a little entente later in the day.
Medical School was not without some humour.
Our anatomy demonstrator taught us that students lose their penises through their coital habits – the mnemonic of the era for the wrist bones: Scaphoid Lunate, Triquetral, Pisiform, Trapezium. Trapezoid, Capitate, Hamate. This was thus imparted to the three chaps at the dissecting table: "I'm going for a cup of coffee now; I expect the (three) girls also to know it when I get back". Good chap.
I too recall Prof. Scothorne – a remarkable man who could draw on the green (yes, I think it was green) board, from memory as well as an amazing comprehension, a cross-section of a curled-up foetus in any plane at any stage of development over 8 months or more.
Just to think of that expertise now fills me with admiration.

He was also extremely and disquietingly observant. "Ah, the arrow that flyeth in the dark striketh!" said he, when he had asked a question of the only one of 96 students who had not attended his previous lecture – and the unfortunate chap could not answer other than to say meekly, "I'm sorry Sir, I missed the last lecture." Guess who the chap was.

In our later years of training, we were farmed out to hospitals of our choosing around the world to broaden our experiences. The above-described, elective period adrenaline fuelled end-of-life simulatory experience was considerably softened by the presence of a young Grecian - Maria Anagnostopolou who was there, in Downpatrick, undertaking her voluntary service, although unfortunately chaperoned by the much less attractive Rita whose ever-presence was a considerable draw-back – but also by a successive Margaret, Maria and Marit – who completed the 4Ms of the 6-week sojourn in the Emerald Isle. Keith Baxby has some knowledge of the above.

I recall the trek up Slieve Donard mentioned by Keith, and also being left in charge of the Hospital one night when the only admission was a young lad with a ruptured appendix. I still recall with a lingering anxiety the relief when the surgical registrar who had to be summoned from Belfast to see to him was in agreement with my diagnosis and undertook the subsequent life-saving laparotomy.

To counterbalance the above success, my suturing of the thin skin over the shin bone of another Casualty who attended the hospital had a much less satisfactory outcome when the wound broke down – as I now know they usually do when stitched so inexpertly.

Obstetrics was an education and a half. The Registrar rushed into the delivery Suite and said that his colleague thought there might be twins. Not possible, declared the hands-on delivering doctor. He was just too late to catch the second baby as it was expelled and dangled at the end of the umbilical cord. Baby survived and was fine.

Less fine was the mother in labour with her legs in stirrups who could see nothing of the manipulations beyond the green sheets covering the stirrups and her legs, though doubtless knew of the presence of a few of us learning the trade beyond the drapes.

We each had to clock up twenty deliveries during our stay at the Maternity Hospital and one of our number was designated to chalk this one up.

He was prepared, gowned, gloved and ready at the shoulder of the midwife in charge. After a prolonged second stage of labour, the midwife said, loud enough for all to hear: "I'm afraid you're going to lose this one (one to chalk up towards your 20) love". I shall never forget the scream from the mother on hearing that she was about to lose her baby. All was put as right as it could be, of course, and the baby was fine – but another vital lesson learned, hugely traumatic for the poor lass involved.

Briefly, my career initially included the intention to be a surgeon, abruptly abandoned to become an NHS Family Doctor in West Yorkshire for 9 years, overlapping with a role as Police Surgeon and a transition to non-NHS General Practice for the remaining 37 years of active working life.

Qualifying, and proceeding Dunelm (Durham) rather than Newcastle, resulted in two disparate comments from our mentors. Henry Miller shook my hand and said, "Well, you bugger, you've done it!". Peter Turney, Consultant Surgeon from Whitehaven, under whose care and tutelage I sojourned for many weeks, wrote to me and included the comment "…. Now you have a licence to learn." How very, very true – and something I have had innumerable opportunities to recall in the last five decades.

Surgical housemanship with Ken Wilson as my Chief in Halifax was thoroughly rewarding and instructive. He was the epitome of sincerity, care, professionalism. I was the only white doctor under Consultant status, which proved a slight difficulty when I phoned a local GP at 0100 hours at a time when I was full of righteous indignation. He had caused me to be taken out of theatre where Ken and I were undertaking a nephrectomy.

The urgent admission was for a man who had called his doctor to complain of severe upper abdominal pain. The pressed or lazy GP had made a telephone diagnosis of a perforated duodenal ulcer. Such confidence in remote diagnostic ability justifying emergency ambulances has always eluded me.

The patient jumped on the bed as I approached and told me that he was feeling well again. No, his doctor hadn't visited him, but just told him that he would send him to hospital in an Ambulance.

I was incandescent at being hauled out of an operation for such an inconsiderate admission and the indigestion-suffering patient was soon on his way home – albeit under his own steam.

Later, my early-hours call to the GP to report on his acute admission had had to be in my best "Indian" accent (for a reason hinted at above). Later that day, I was the only surgical team colleague who wasn't questioned by the aptly named hospital Manager, Willy Weeks, as to whether or not he had been the one to rouse the hapless doctor with a long, rambling progress report on his patient. My fellow housemen were in stitches. I confessed, arrogantly justifying my early hours communication with the GP, not long returned from his honeymoon.

Two of the other surgeons were, I understood, elderly former GPs who had been drafted into surgery at the beginning of the second world war. One baulked at an early morning procedure which I had conscientiously arranged as an emergency for the removal of a blood clot from the left brachial artery of a poor chap who had had unnecessary varicose vein surgery (yes, we couldn't easily work out the anatomy of the connection between the two pathologies). The surgeon procrastinated for a fortnight and, after above elbow amputation the poor chap eventually succumbed and left hospital in a coffin.

The other surgeon did only two ward rounds in 6 months. One of the two diagnoses he made was "Nonsense – appendicitis – get it out". The Registrar and I were aghast and sent the man home forthwith to recover from his gastritis. On the other occasion he was undertaking an (arguably unnecessary even in those days) Gritti-Stokes left knee amputation when the anaesthetist called urgently for blood. I had had it ready in defiance of an order that it wasn't necessary and met with opprobrium from the disgruntled surgeon as we changed post-operatively. "When are you leaving?" *"In about a fortnight"*. "It won't be too soon." Damn it - and him; I had saved his bacon.

The 13-year-old mature girl with right-sided lower abdominal pain, but normal blood readings, languished for a week on the Ward until my registrar told me to take her appendix out.

I argued that she was not suffering from appendicitis, but he prevailed. She had said that …. "Dad's a bastard, gets drunk, beats us up and life is pretty horrible at home". The appendix was visually and histologically normal. She recovered fully.

However, the same day as her operation, her 11-year-old brother was admitted with LIF (left lower abdominal) pain without any clinical indications on offer – which was not appendicitis either clinically or in the textbooks.

He concurred: Dad's a bastard etc etc. Blood tests were normal, and he was put to bed for the night. Next morning, he was very hot and had right-sided abdominal pain with rebound tenderness; I removed his gangrenous appendix.

Thereafter, there were no more appendix stories to relate and the lesson - which could have been designed as an exam question or study - was well learned and has stood me in good stead ever since.

Perhaps it was stretching things a little when a young man with abdominal pain was under my care many years later. His surgery involved a quadruple pathology. We removed a six-inch (15cm) long appendix which had migrated from the right to the left side of the abdomen, excised an inflamed appendix epiploica (the actual cause of his malaise) and took the opportunity, on the "way out" to correct his Meckel's diverticulum and repair his umbilical hernia. Four for the price of one.

Medicine under Dr Chris Davidson in Bradford (Chris was doubly qualified in Medicine and Dentistry) was a sleepless delight. The four GPs who visited the Ward during my 6-month spell there had very differing reasons for pleading with me to join their Practices. One, a West Indian charmer said that their aim was to work just 20 hours per week; another (who was known for pocketing the packet of fags from the bar counter at the drug Company free lunches) told me that they could just do with another young Jewish lad in the Practice. But I am not Jewish. A third didn't inspire me, but a fourth did and I switched from thoughts of surgery to the excitement of joining a four-man Practice where the prospects of a fulfilling life in the Community beckoned – with two of my partners-to-be nearing retirement.

GENERAL PRACTICE REALISATIONS

It was the first week of my life on the front line in General Practice. Mr M.I. came in supported physically, emotionally and possibly in other ways too, by his male companion.

The back pain was "very, very bad – too much bad, tacleef, tacleef, I'm telling you".

Examination gave no clues.

Probably inappropriate, by todays' standards, treatment was prescribed and a one-week certificate for time off work provided.

But "He need two week, doctor."

"Not in the first instance; if he……. "He need two week, doctor."

"One week to see how he goes, then come back for assessme…..……..". "He really need two week, doctor." More lingua franca, unintelligible to me.
Guns were metaphorically adhered to and he left the surgery (tacleef, tacleef), limping and supported even more by his companion.
I watched as he left the premises but, by the end of the drive, he was walking normally.
I fumed on the spot, having been duped, though not quite as badly had the "two-weeker" been given.
Chasing after him in the car, stopping, screeching alongside, I jumped out and snatched the certificate and prescription from his hand, with a few words of advice on cheating and fraud.
"But he need two-week……………"
Perhaps the visit to Pakistan for the two-week wedding celebrations would have to be taken as holiday rather than "on the sick".
I never found out – nor did I care.
*
0720. It's urgent: she's in real bad pain. Can you come and see her? Yes, of course. Are you coming now? I'm just getting dressed: How long has she had it? Is this the first…….But are you coming now? …. Yes…Is she bleeding? You are coming, aren't you? Yes, five minutes………
I helped her from toilet to bed and advised that the birth of her baby was imminent, and I would get her into hospital………. "What baby?" Oops.
Neither she, her mother, father, boyfriend, sister (who had three children) was aware of the pregnancy – and she was not an overweight girl. Later in the day, I popped in to see her.
How are you now?..........Oh, fine thank you Doctor………. And how is baby?...........What baby?
It is hard to imagine her state of mind and such a shame that she could not have realised her gravid state sooner in order to have had received comprehensive ante-natal care. None of my partners knew of the pregnancy. And it was not the only occasion we had the same scenario in the Practice.
On another occasion and in another setting, a 15-year-old had given birth on her own in her bedroom. The mattress was soaked in blood. Two weeks later she was toxic and admitted to hospital. The dead baby was found in and retrieved from a box in the wardrobe.

I was asked to confirm life extinct. What a crying shame. What an unspeakable tragedy that she could not confide in her mum. Even in this enlightened age we come across similar problems – to our collective shame.

"I've got to see the doctor today." .... "*OK: 1015 then.*"
.... "I can't come then."

No, of course not: last orders are at 1030.

Wednesday afternoon surgeries in those days ran from 4 pm with appointments every 5 minutes.

A near neighbour – who I did know as one of the Practice patients was of a nervous disposition and afeared of hospitals. The huge melon sized testicular hydrocoele was an encumbrance too far, ".... but I wouldn't be able to have an operation doctor......well I would if it could be done without warning.... No, I couldn't.... I'll put up with it......if it could just be removed without me knowing...."

Sunday evening: I called the on-duty Senior Surgical Registrar....
" .... Are you busy?

"No, not really" ....

"Fancy something different?"

The impending patient's wife was in on the deal. He was on the table within the hour and job (marsupialisation) done in short order. His wife was delighted. He wasn't! I don't think he forgave me for doing his bidding. Or perhaps he did, but just couldn't admit it to me. Such an arrangement is unthinkable nowadays. Perhaps he had another agenda of which I was never aware.

In the early seventies' 'flu epidemics, one day resulted in two surgeries of 20 patients each and 49 home visits. Of the 90 presenting with flu-like or flu-actual symptoms, one seemed more ill than the others and she was admitted to hospital that day.

She was soon diagnosed with TB meningitis – and recovered. I was arguably possibly less astute on another occasion with the lady complaining of indigestion; she rounded on me one day to point out that I had failed to diagnose her leukaemia on presentation. Mea culpa.

Lawrence, Heavy-weight boxer Richard Dunn's trainer, said "Bloody 'ell, you're worse 'n me!" when, on crutches, with a left leg in plaster after fracturing the 5th metatarsal a day or two earlier, I visited him to assess his painful foot.

A few weeks later I met his wife out shopping: "How's Lawrence? "Oh, he's not right good, but he says he can't see you after you visited him and were worse than him, doctor."

Richard used to ask me to go out running with him – but I didn't dare embarrass myself.

The GP stories are, of course endless – some triumphant, some tragic, others humbling and yet others which cause one to blush at diagnostic failures.

Police work was also absorbing – some 20,000 cases seen in 2 years. The false plaster cast on a snitch - for the Regional Crime Squad – then the gang fractured his arm as a punishment.

The Yorkshire Ripper. Although I saw his victims, I only saw him for a drink-driving offence.

Dec 6, 1974 - Piper Navajo Crash – all 10 dead near Leeds Bradford Airport

(The twin engine airplane departed Leeds-Bradford Airport at 1715LT on a charter flight to Staverton, carrying a pilot and seven employees of the ICI Fibres Company. During initial climb in marginal weather conditions, the airplane encountered difficulties then control was lost. It entered a dive and crashed in a field located two miles from the airport. The aircraft was destroyed, and all eight occupants were killed. The accident occurred six minutes after take-off.

FORENSICE AND PSEUDO-FORENSICS

I was not often in the Lake District on a Saturday afternoon, but 15th May 1985 was an exception. The mobile 'phone conversation with HM Coroner James Turnbull resulted in my being in Bradford an hour or so later.

The Police Escort from The Lakes did not catch up with me in my trusty Honda Accord, so a car from Bradford was despatched and we met somewhere near Kildwick in a sort of relay manoeuvre where I relinquished the spearhead for the remainder of the journey.

My brief was to extricate the bodies from Bradford City Football Stadium – and to achieve it before dawn, if possible, so as to limit rubber-necking which it was assumed was bound, after dawn, to be an unwanted accompaniment to our endeavours. I called upon long term colleagues, former Newcastle graduates who were local Police Surgeons, to assist. Together, working through the night, we completed the task.

Many of the bodies were burned to a cinder, dentition substantially excepted, welded to the ground in the melted roof materials which by then had enveloped them. The Chief Constable, Colin Sampson, was on the scene for a while and was surprised that the only facilities I asked for were some shovels, picks and new dustbins – into which we shovelled everything within a reasonable distance of each body, with forensics in mind. We retrieved 52 bodies, many incomplete, though we no doubt had the missing limbs and other cindered parts in our bins.

On two occasions I had to break off to advise in respect of distressed Police Officers. One, working on his hands and knees was hoping or dreading to find a cousin who he believed to be amongst the victims. Another was in floods of tears at the enormity of the task and the dead. Both were gently relieved of their duties.

The following day I spent five minutes in the stadium alone with Margaret Thatcher who was deeply moved. It was special to have that brief time with her and to sense the depth of her compassion and concern.

Dental records solved identification problems.

THE CHIMNEY

It was one of the saddest of call-outs to confirm death in a very young infant. Always discussing such tragic deaths with a Home Office Pathologist, I called in at the City Mortuary to see Professor David Gee. He was undertaking a post-mortem examination on the body of a man. We discussed my child and agreed that there was no indication for further Police action just then, but a post-mortem would be conducted as a matter of routine.

Whilst there, two detectives also called in – bearing three severed limbs found on a local tip. It turned out that they were amputations from a Leeds Hospital where the limbs had been transported to the wrong disposal facility.

But the man on the table was there because of an inability to stop blow-back of fumes from a gas fire in an office near the city Centre. The dehydrated, mummified body was extricated from the chimney flue and it was deduced that he had been there for a few decades as his pockets contained a 1D (one penny in old money) bus ticket of the kind that had been out of use for some time. It seems that he had been hiding from someone or got stuck or died in the course of an attempt to enter the premises via the chimney.

I never got to hear the full story.

CITY CENTRE FACILITY – JOINED UP MEDICINE/SURGERY

The senior surgeon and I were just finishing an elective procedure and conversation turned to the events of the previous week. What had I been doing in the forensic field?

I recounted the finding by a member of the public of an umbilical cord hanging over the rim of a ladies' toilet in the Centre of the City. My job was to decide if it could be human or otherwise. It had the characteristics of bowel and lacked the three vessel-component to be of the suspected origin. The pathologist concurred.

The surgeon could help with new information. That same day they had admitted a man who told how, in order to relieve his constipation, he had stuck a knife into his perineum and extracted a long segment of bowel which he had then cut off. As this made him feel unwell, he decided to seek help at the local hospital; he got on a bus for the mile or so ride to the Casualty Unit – and was admitted for reconstruction and referral to the mental health services.

PERSONAL MEDICAL AFFLICTIONS AFFECTING WORK

I have been fortunate beyond belief to have had only 4-5 days off work in the last 55 years but being on the other side of the counter is instructive.

In our student days I decided to demolish my old Morris Minor RGT 66.

The left upper arm injury caused by carelessness swinging a sledgehammer and impaling my left upper arm on a jagged sheet door strut caused an internal bleed which compressed the left radial nerve and I had first-hand instruction in the effects of wrist drop.

As it was approaching "Last orders" time at the Brandling, Chris Lynch and I pondered only briefly and concluded that we should detour on our way to Casualty in order to get a bevy in. This decision was not the best I have ever made prior to the inevitable requirement for surgery and resulted in the difficult question ("When did you last have anything to eat or drink?" Er…….) a short while later in the RVI when the decision was to give me a general anaesthetic to explore the wound in order to stem the bleeding and relieve the compression on the nerve which was giving me "Saturday night paralysis".

So-called because of its prevalence amongst young lovers with arms around their girls in the back row of the cinema. (Always most debilitating when bilateral after swapping sides to alleviate the effects on the first arm).
The subsequent procedure under local anaesthetic is best described as horrible, but the lesson was well learned.
After this trauma, in the early hours, Chris and I decided that it was too late to go back to our respective lodgings, so popped over to the Lake District in his Morris 1100, BBR 75C, to enjoy the tranquillity of the roads. He drove there and I drove back with the benefit of him changing gear for me in the joint driving effort which we dubbed "thinkromesh" – by virtue of me dipping the clutch and he having intuitive knowledge of the gear to which I wished to be transferred. As the trip progressed, he became adept at changing the gear without any conversation or clutch operation, but simply on application or release of the accelerator. For some unaccountable reason, this technique has not become a feature of standard instructions in Driving Academies.
The chest infection as a houseman resulted in my being sent off the Ward for a few hours and overnight.
Right acromionectomy was done one Saturday morning, but not helped by the well-meaning discharge nurse who clapped me on the operated shoulder in a gesture of good wishes and affection as I was discharged the same morning. I sold the non-power-steering Porsche 944 with only 1066 miles on the clock.
The Septoplasty was undertaken one late Good Friday afternoon after I had seen three of my flock into theatre for surgery before I was due on the table. Having the interminably long nasal ribbon packs removed the following morning was about as excruciating a few minutes as I can ever remember; the worst of it is that after one has been extracted, there is still one to go! The idea of the procedure having been booked for a Good Friday was to minimise incoming calls from patients. It didn't work. There were 32 of them in 72 hours. On the way home from surgery the next morning I saw a poorly bairn and talked someone else through suicidal ideas and out the other side of their problem. Anaesthetic and brain fog are the probable reasons for my forgetting details of the remainder of the weekend's problems.
Left ulnar nerve release at the elbow under a regional anaesthetic was a joy because we were able to chat throughout.

Only a partial success; it would merit transposition (re-routing to the layman).

A slicing injury to the left middle finger-tip was in effect a guillotine injury between two heavy packs of kitchen tiles. My surgeon colleague thought that I would lose the last phalanx of the finger, but I persuaded him that a few stitches would save the day – and in any event I had a Chunnel train to catch for the 777-mile trip by road to France that afternoon, driving a manual Mercedes Vito with a trailer and two tons of tiles distributed between car and trailer. I promised him that I would keep the hand elevated above the heart for the whole of the 15-hour trip – and did so, changing gear with my right hand as I had practised in student days before Chris Lynch and I applied thinkromesh in BBR 75C.

An emergency stop in the car on the third post-operative day for right knee surgery was accomplished with initial ease, but such early return behind the wheel is not to be recommended for reasons which are clearer in retrospect than in anticipation.

DELUSIONS

One of the toughest Police Officers I have ever come across was severely injured in a road accident and eventually invalided out of the Force.

His general medical care had been without further major incident for many years, but, after some time becoming increasingly more introverted, he developed the fixed delusion that he had hairs up to three feet long growing from most of his body. Many hours of consultation were spent in trying to understand this and his avoidance techniques for others seeing him in what he had sufficient insight to realise was an unusual attribute, but he left my care to seek to persuade other doctors of his extraordinary affliction and I have never heard further from him.

A middle-aged man – who I had never seen before (common in a multi-thousand list Practice) was suicidal and I was called to see him at home. He had been sexually involved with a 13-year old girl, and was full of fear and remorse at the impending legal proceedings. He had been to the Public Library to suss-out how much Valium he would need to end it all painlessly and quickly.

Hey, not so fast! What other medication are you taking? Amongst other things – Madopar. For how long? Just a few weeks.

To cut a long story short, withdrawal of the Madopar resulted in compete resolution of his delusion and his believed reason for his impending suicide. It had all been in his mind. Another salutary tale.

GETTING ABOUT

Although based in Yorkshire, I did seem to get around a bit in the 45 years or so in General Practice. In the early '70s I had nine separate weeks at The Institutes for the Achievement of Human Potential, run by Glenn Doman, remedial Physiotherapist in Chestnut Hill, Pennsylvania. I am not sure even now if there was great overall benefit either to the brain-compromised children I accompanied there – or to my fund of knowledge, but it was certainly rewarding to meet and get to know many others interested in their work and to indulge in a passion for flying – often on the flight-decks of Boeing 747s; dropping into JFK hard on the heels of a Tristar is a wonderful experience…….

My incidental, usually on the spur of the moment, journeys took me to Gibraltar for an hour in order to bring home a mother and newborn light birth-weight baby, to London on several occasions for urgent cranial surgery, to London again for cardiomyopathy leading later to a Glasgow to Manchester dash for heart transplant surgery, to Monaco for cardiac catheterisation and stent insertion, Edinburgh in the early days of percutaneous nephrolithotomy.

Hong Kong to bring home a young lady with a gynae problem, a dash by air to Cornwall for a psychological upheaval, Ulverston four times in 36 hours for a cancer-denial and urgent amputation problem, Newcastle upon Tyne for a rare seizure problem, Liverpool for cardiac issues, Lanzarote for stroke and treatment issues, Wrexham for stroke problems, Boston USA for cryogenic discussions, Peterborough for a bicycle accident/fractured hip, Detroit for a television interview, Chur in Switzerland for pancreatitis, Broze in Gaillac for a (baby) delivery, St Jean Cap Ferrat for cardiac issues, Hereford for medical equipment, Brisbane Australia, Lockerbie after the Pan Am crash to confirm dozens of deaths and on many more occasions over the ensuing week.

Over one twenty-year-period I drove some 40,000 miles per year, day and night, in and around West Yorkshire checking human remains, remains thought to be human which turned out to be sheep or other animal bones.

Dealing with psychiatric emergencies, murder, multiple murders, accidental terminal shootings, other accidental deaths on hillsides, in forests, in quarries, rape, child abuse, suicide, critical road accidents, people trapped in all manner of vehicles, headless bodies on railway lines – to mention but a few.

On one occasion I went for an "Experiential Weekend" (training, I hasten to add) in London only to leave at the end of the first day as I could not get the message. On another occasion I had three engagements in London on the same day – at a time when I hadn't been there for many years – at Winthrop Laboratories, Browns Hotel and The Guildhall – returning home the same day.

On the afternoon my Cessna 152, which I had sold to the local Flying School, was crashed, I was flown up to Teesside to encourage the newly paraplegic flying Instructor to have surgery to stabilise his spine so as to aid his mobilisation. Then I was flown back again to "do" the evening surgery. Following which I was flown North again to assist with the surgery. Thence home. All in a day's work.

I have met and had interesting discussions with the Yorkshire Ripper (for a drink-drive offence), George Bush Senior (unmemorable chat), Archbishop Desmond Tutu (to find we had had a mutual acquaintance in Father Trevor Huddlestone who wrote "Naught for your Comfort" and predicted the heinous, tragic events in Soweto). Professor Raymond Dart (who discovered Australopithicus africanus), Francis Crick (of double helix of DNA fame), Gazza with a leg in pot, Stephanie Powers, Mikhail Gorbachev (who was charming and spoke in Russian via an interpreter and Latin without an interpreter!), Colin Powell (who told us how he had filled in his swimming pool to stop the children abusing it), Margaret Thatcher (who was touched when she attended the Bradford Football stadium fire scene) and Tony Blair (who said "Oh yes….." when I gave him my name). I kept in touch with Lord Walton right up to his Green College days. I have the fond memory of sharing experiences with the recently deceased Murray Walker; what a privilege to have done so.

Do I wish I had travelled any route other than the medical highway? Not on your Nellie.

Would I do it all again? At the drop of a hat, but with a rejuvenated chassis, engine and gearbox, of course. But I would now know what I did not know the first time round and it could make a difference.

Peter Irvin

Sod's Law

Many years ago, before the days of mobile phones, a good GP friend, who was Police Surgeon for the area, had some pressing engagement which would take him out of the area for a short while. He asked me if I would cover him for an hour and reassured me that the chances of anything happening "were miniscule."

Ten minutes into the hour that I was covering, the phone rang and, yes, it was the Police! (Sod's Law in all its glory.) Could I go down to the Police Station where they were dealing with a murder case!! (Sod's Law squared) On arrival, I was taken down to the cells and introduced to a scruffy, long haired youth who was the suspected murderer.

My job, I was told, was to take a sample of his hair and I was given a pair of surgical gloves and a pair of scissors. I was advised to take a sample from a place that would not leave him looking like someone who had been attacked by a very amateur barber, so I took half an inch from underneath the back of his greasy mullet and carefully placed it in a plastic bag. And that was it. Never heard any more about the case. No commendations for the part that I played.

As I drove home, I thought that they had been exceptionally lucky to have someone with my (very modest) surgical skills to perform such a delicate procedure. When I got home the hour was up. I reckon that I probably hold the World Record for involvement in incidents, PER HOUR ON DUTY, for Police Surgeons.

A Ferry Trip to Holland

We had just got onto the Hull to Rotterdam ferry on our way to Germany to see our daughter. A week of peace beckoned. We left our cabin and headed to the bar and by now the ferry was well down the Humber estuary. I was about a third of the way down my beer when I heard, over the loudspeaker, the words I always dread, "Is there a doctor on the ship?"

I made my way to the Purser's Office and announced that I was, indeed, a doctor and the Purser looked mightily relieved. I was informed that there was a chap on board with chest pains. He was one of several hundred veterans of the Second World War, all in their seventies and eighties, who were on their way over to an anniversary meeting in Holland.

The Purser told me that a few months earlier the ship had been full of veterans going to some other anniversary and there had been several deaths during the crossing. Had there been no doctor on board today then the Purser himself would have had no choice but to turn the ship around and head back to Hull. There was no medical equipment on board, and I had not brought any along as I was on holiday. I was led down into the bowels of the ship and there I met Sid.

Sid, 77 years old and from Lincolnshire, told me that he did suffer with angina and he had his GTN spray, which usually gave him relief whenever he got the pain. However, today, the pain was easing only slightly and not as quickly as usual, despite having used it several times. His pulse, colour and breathing were all fine, but he looked very tired. The Purser then informed me, in front of Sid, that I must make the decision as to whether the ship turned round and went back to Hull. At this point Sid miraculously rallied. He informed me in no uncertain terms that he was NOT going back. He had waited years for this opportunity to go over to Holland with his pals and he was going on, even if it killed him.

What could I do? A patient with known IHD whose chest pain was not responding to GTN would normally, on dry land, be whisked to the local hospital but here, heading out into the North Sea, things were different. I thought long and hard and he did seem a little stronger than he was when I had entered the cabin. He told me that the pain was easing off but whether he was being truthful I was not sure. I sat and chatted to him for a while and he eventually told me that the pain had gone. But had it really? He was determined that he was going on and that nothing was going to stop him, and I suppose it could well have been that this reunion with his old comrades was one of the few meaningful things left in his lifetime. I just couldn't bring myself to have him sent back home and wondered if the act of sending him back might kill him! We agreed that I would go back and see him in thirty minutes and when I saw him again, he seemed fine. I went back to see him on two further occasions that evening and, again, he seemed well enough.

I told the Purser to let me know if there were any problems in the night, but I was not disturbed. I saw Sid the next morning and he was very bright and looking forward to his onward trip. He thanked me profusely, although in reality I had done very little other than reassure him, and kept my fingers crossed.

On docking, the veterans were being met by medical teams, so I felt a lot easier about him. I last saw him disembarking with some of his pals and he looked happy and well.
Kathy and I were lucky in one sense. On booking our crossing, because of the number of veterans that had pre-booked, we had been told that there were no cabins available with their own shower and we were not looking forward to using communal facilities. However, after my dealings with Sid an en suite cabin mysteriously appeared at no extra cost, as did a bottle of wine at our evening meal.
Good old Sid. I don't know what would have happened if he had not put his foot down and insisted on staying on board. Was he lying about the pain easing? I will, of course, never know. I may well have had to turn the ship around.
What a decision that would have been.

A Relative Revelation

The only member of my extended family who had ever had any connection to the medical profession was a great uncle who had been an orderly in the Medical Corps in WW1. A fairly tenuous link, but my mother was convinced that it was the reason that I took up medicine, as the great uncle was from her side of the family.
For many years, I was sure that there was no-one else with a medical bent in the family but one day we had a locum in the practice for a couple of days and he said that he thought that he and I might be related. We soon established that our grandmothers were sisters, mine being the first and his being the last, of twelve kids, in the days when families were very large. This nicely explained the age difference between him and me and we decided that it made us second cousins (common great grandparents).
He went on to tell me that he had a brother (also my second cousin, of course) who had two boys who were hoping to go on to Med School, but things were being delayed because they were both very good athletes. "Very good" turned out to be an understatement. They were Alistair and Jonny B. who won gold and bronze at the 2012 London Olympics and gold and silver at the 2016 Rio Olympics, in the Triathlon. They are still competing and are hoping to eventually get back to their medical courses.

I have certainly dined out many times with the story of being related to these two famous athletes and have even suggested, with not a great deal of success, that they got their abilities from being related to me. I hope that, one day, they do qualify in Medicine because that will then make four of us in the family. And, of course, we are all related to Great Uncle Charlie of the WW1 Medical Corps. So maybe my Mum was right, and he was the catalyst that started the whole thing off.

Knysna, South Africa

Sitting in a restaurant outside Knysna, South Africa, the waitress* says, "Are you a doctor?" "Well, yes I am," I reply, somewhat surprised. "Can you help? There's a man in the garden who seems to be ill."

(*In those days and for many years afterwards waiters and waitresses were known, collectively, as waitrons in South Africa. "Hello, Sir, my name is Wayne/Kylie, and I will be your waitron for this evening." It was one of those daft PC things when it was thought that there should be no differentiation between males and females. I always thought that it made them sound like robots. It seems to have died away a lot now, but we still occasionally hear the term.)

It's dusk now and the garden area is deserted apart from a body stretched out on the grass and a man kneeling by his side, holding his wrist in a medical sort of way, presumably checking his pulse. As I approach, he looks up and asks, "Are you a physician?" to which I reply," Yes".

"Thank God for that," he says, "I'm a gynaecologist and have no idea how to deal with this situation. You will need to take over." As I kneel beside the man the gynaecologist walks away, in my mind I'm thinking to get more help. But, no, he's walked away never to be seen again!! Thanks, pal, great if we need to do CPR which back then ideally needed two people. (I'd like to think that not all gynaecologists would react in this way.)

The chap on the lawn is very grey, says he has a heavy pain in his chest, is thick set and is probably in his early sixties. Most likely an M.I. but, luckily, his pulse and breathing are OK. We're about five miles from Knysna and the road to town runs alongside the lagoon so I have a very good view, over the water, of the flashing lights on the ambulance that's on its way.

It arrives soon afterwards, parks up at the front and two "paramedics" arrive at the back-garden area with a stretcher on a wheeled trolley. I use the word paramedics in its very broadest sense because in South Africa, in the eighties, to do this job you only needed to be a big strong lad who, with another big strong lad, could lift very large Afrikaaner patients into an ambulance (and some Afrikaaners are extremely large).

So, they have their trolley on an area that's about twelve inches above the level of the lawn on which our patient is lying. One of them says to the patient, "Come on then, get on the stretcher." I tell them that I'm a medic and point out to them that this man is extremely ill and I think it better that *they* lift him onto the stretcher. With much tutting and sighing they go down onto the lawn and get him onto the stretcher, then onto the trolley, then into the ambulance and off they go.

Job done, I wander back to the restaurant upstairs, watching the flashing lights heading back to town and hoping that he makes it. My wife and fellow diners have had my main course taken away to be kept warm but it's not particularly warm and they had all finished eating, so the enjoyment of the meal is almost gone. We consoled ourselves with more wine.

I collared the waitress and asked her how she knew that I was a doctor. It wasn't as though I had a stethoscope around my neck. She said, "Well, you just looked like one." To this very day I have never known what a doctor looks like. I've met all shapes and sizes, various degrees of sartorial elegance or otherwise and could never, in a million years, pick out a doctor in a crowd.

But the South African waitress did.

High Tech 0 Simplicity 1

It had been a routine BP check and contained no surprises. For once, I was on time with my appointments when I heard the phrase beloved by GPs, "While I'm here, Doctor….."

The patient, a 54 year old steelworker, told me that he had a lump on his chest which had been present for about three months and his wife had insisted that he mention it today (he obviously had no choice then).

I expected that it would be the usual knobbly costosternal joint or prominent xiphisternum but when he took off his shirt there it was – a lump about 10 cm across sitting over the third rib and about 5cm to the right of the sternum. It was very firm, rose in the centre to a peak but had no definite edge. It was not at all tender, seemed very much fixed in position and it was hard to tell whether it originated in the skin or the rib. He had not lost any weight, had no other symptoms and I could find nothing else on examination. Some sort of cyst or something more sinister?

It obviously needed further investigation without too much delay, but I now had the problem of deciding to which department I should refer him. Dermatology, Orthopaedics or even Cardiothoracic? I finally opted for General Surgery, mainly because waiting times for the others were usually so incredibly long and I knew the surgeon pretty well.

He was seen within two weeks and the surgeon was fairly certain that it was either an osteochondroma or an osteosarcoma. He was taken onto the ward for X-rays and "probable radiotherapy." Xray suggested a chondrosarcoma, bone scan showed "increased uptake." CT scan stated, "the main tumour mass is in the anterior end of the third rib, there is bony destruction, pleural changes and invasion of the muscles of the anterior chest wall." There seemed to be" enlarged retrosternal and right para-tracheal nodes but no metastases in the lungs."

Biopsy was performed and histology showed "striated muscle bundles within collagenous connective tissue, chronic inflammatory cell infiltrate but no evidence of neoplasia."

So, after all this high-tech investigation there was still no definitive diagnosis and the surgeon referred him on to the Cardiothoracic department where the consultant felt that it was a chondrosarcoma and needed excision.

Before surgery the patient was shown to have normal pulmonary function, normal FBC and LFTs and there was no paraprotein detected. At operation there was swollen costal cartilage which laterally appeared necrotic and there were adhesions between cartilage and pleura.

Another biopsy, frozen section, was sent off but gave no clear indication as to the histology so the anterior ends of the second and third ribs along with their costal cartilages were removed and a Silastic mesh put in place.

So, we've now had high tech investigations and surgery with frozen section and we still don't know what this is. Someone then, apparently, decided to see if there was any bacterial activity in the excised mass and sent it off to Bacteriology. And what did they grow on the Petri dish – Salmonella!! The chest wound began to discharge and a swab showed...... Salmonella!! At last, a diagnosis – Salmonella Osteomyelitis. The simplest test, culture, had given us the answer.

The wound continued to discharge for a few weeks but eventually dried up and healed after an extended course of co-trimoxazole. Success at last. We were, of course, too optimistic because six months later he returned and showed me a lump on the left side of his chest – a perfect mirror image of the original and sitting over the left third rib, 5cm to the left of the sternum!! It all seemed rather surreal.

The cardiothoracic surgeon felt that we should try medical treatment first, rather than more surgery, and he started on a nine-week course of pivmecillinam which caused the mass to subside. Despite having no further antibiotics, the mass completely disappeared after another three months. I saw him regularly over the years for his BP checks and usually had a quick peep at his chest just to make sure there was no recurrence. There never was. I had never seen a case before and have never seen one since but could I have been one of the few GPs in the country, on seeing an unusual lump, to include Salmonella Osteomyelitis in his list of differential diagnoses?

Bribery and Corruption?

It's 17 years since I saw a pharmaceutical rep but I'm still, to this day, using pens that they gave me. How relationships with drug companies changed between beginning in General Practice and ending. The earlier days involved gifts of tape recorders, very basic computers, calculators (which were something special then), various other electronic gadgets and, of course, pens. But then, on top of that, were the lavish trips out to five star restaurants and plush hotels along with our wives. And, if you were a golfer, and the rep just happened to play golf too, we got trips to many local courses and sometimes to smart, famous golf courses around the country.

I knew some GPs who had trips to Europe from various companies, but I obviously didn't prescribe enough of their products.

I remember golf trips to Slaley Hall, The Belfry and Turnberry (now called Trump Turnberry, with room only now starting at £179 per night) for two night stays and at least one round of golf with all food and drinks included. But no wives, which was very sensible amongst a gang of golfers, simply because, in general, I've found that wives don't understand golf. Of course, I didn't particularly go for the golf, the food or the sumptuous hotel but it was just that I found that the gentle reminder about the efficacy of Ibuprofamoxyfrusebendroneomycin and its almost total lack of side effects seemed to be much more deeply instilled into my brain than having the same chat in my surgery.

At one of the above-mentioned golf courses, I remember the first evening, after a superb meal, being no less than a riotous drinkfest and can only vaguely recall staggering up to my room. Next thing I knew it was morning, I was fully clothed, lying across the top of the bedclothes with the room lights on. I had been in a coma for eight hours. I had to then force down breakfast and go out and play golf, very difficult with a huge hangover. Then in the afternoon attend a lecture about Ibuprofamoxyfrusebendroneomycin and how it was so much more effective than its rivals. We all drank a lot less on the second evening.

Then things changed. I still remember with great clarity the day a rep came in and announced that pharmaceutical regulations had changed and that, shock, horror, they were only allowed to dish out gifts worth £5 or less. He said that the best they could do was an umbrella because they could bulk purchase them for £4.99. We still got the pen though. So everything changed overnight – no more gadgetry, no gourmet evenings and certainly no more golf tournaments. I was stunned and almost had to take the rest of the day off.

By a strange coincidence, it was just about this time that I had started to think about not taking gifts from reps anymore as I had begun to feel quite guilty about the possibility that I was being bribed. So, following that I only saw reps that I actually liked, probably less than 50% of them.

I think that, morally, I did the right thing.

It's a Dog's Life

Our Old English Sheepdog, Hugo, was 11 years old when he collapsed on the beach. He didn't move at all and we all thought he was dead. Our girls were in tears. Then, after what seemed like forever, he stirred and then slowly stood up. He started moving around and then running. This was a great relief as the car was over half a mile away and I didn't fancy carrying him; he was not a lightweight.

I took him to the Vet who thought he was in cardiac failure and felt that the collapse may have been due to an MI. He thought that the dog should be started on Digoxin, "125 mg, once a day," he said. I was amazed and wondered if dogs metabolized Digoxin in a completely different way to humans and needed 1000 times the human dose. I pointed out that the dose in humans was usually 0.125 mg daily. He looked completely bewildered, "are you sure?" he said. Whilst we were having this conversation, he had reached up to the shelf and grabbed a container of Digoxin tablets and had already counted out thirty of them and had them in a bottle for me. He looked at the container very carefully and said, "Well, well, you're right, these are 0.125 mg after all." He admitted that he had always thought that the dose was 125 mg having got used to simply calling them Digoxin 125. He had been doing this for almost 20 years!!

On the way out I was presented with a bill and, as well as the consultation fee, there was a charge for the Digoxin, £10. Now, I knew that Digoxin was dirt cheap so, when more were required, I popped round to our local, friendly pharmacist and we came to an arrangement. Hugo picked up very quickly and was back to normal in no time. He lived for another two years to an age that was quite unusual for the breed.

New Tech, Savings and Efficiency

Way back when, when computers were in their infancy, we had a meeting with the FPC, as it was then known. Not sure what it’s called now but “progress” always involves changing names. They suggested that we start thinking about the use of computers in the Practice. We were totally computer illiterate at the time, but they gradually convinced us that, once installed and running, we would be able to employ less staff, become more efficient and, therefore, save money.

So, with a bit of help from a computer buff friend of mine we acquired a single computer with a fairly simple programme, designed by a GP, that stored basic info about the patients. The FPC seemed very pleased with it but within a year they informed us that our self-sourced software was not high tech enough and we must use software of which they approved. Within another couple of months, the PC itself was deemed to be inadequate and we must only use other, more expensive hardware. So, our original hardware and software were ditched and we "moved forward" with more sophisticated gear. Gradually, we increased the number of PCs and, gradually, sometimes with great difficulty, we all learned how to use them.

As time went by, like all practices, we ended up with many PCs throughout the building. The FPC kept in touch and eventually, one day, told us that all the hardware needed to be replaced, as the old stuff just wasn't up to running the new software that they were about to introduce. But we need not worry, because they would pay for all the replacement PCs and we could keep all the old ones for personal use. Win-win situation for us we thought.

Well, not quite. Part of the deal involved the practice signing a contract to have all the new software regularly updated and all the new hardware regularly "maintained" by a company selected by the FPC. This started with a fairly modest monthly payment but as time went by the monthly payments began to escalate, not quite exponentially but by considerably more than inflation. And we couldn't switch to another company as we were tied in by contract.

A couple of years later I realised that we had two, new, full time staff who were solely involved with running the computers and really hefty, monthly maintenance fees for the computer upkeep.

Employing less staff and saving money? Hmmmmmmm.........

It's always said that if something sounds too good to be true then it usually is.

It was.

Some Interesting Home Visits

In my early days in General Practice anyone who asked for a home visit got one: no questions asked. It was not unusual to leave the morning surgery with ten to twelve visits each and there were three of us.

Mondays were the worst days and it got easier as the week went on. Part of the reason, I'm sure, was the fact that we really didn't have enough surgery appointments throughout the day and when we increased them years later the number of visits duly reduced.
I had a few interesting episodes over the years whilst doing home visits. These were the sort of things that never appeared in any of the textbooks.

1. I parked in a street in the old town and went into one of the terraced houses only to find that whilst in there the chimney stack of the adjacent house had collapsed and fallen onto my car. The car roof was extensively damaged but at least it was still driveable. Needless to say, the house owners had no insurance, but I did manage to get it covered by my car insurance but, of course, lost my no claims bonus.
2. I had parked on a fairly narrow road and as I was examining the patient, we all heard a loud bang. Going outside, I found that a large council truck had tried to squeeze past my car and that one of its large wheel nuts had come into contact with my tyre and burst it. The truck driver and his mate helped me change the wheel and off I went. I contacted the Council and they paid for a new tyre.
3. In my early days of home visiting I used to leave my car unlocked when I went into the patient's house – stupid really. I always, of course, took my medical bag with me so there was nothing of any value in the car when I was out of it. On returning to my car after one home visit I found two young boys, aged about five or six, sitting in the two front seats, one of them pretending to drive. They were from the house that I had visited, did no harm whatsoever and jumped out as soon as I arrived. After that I always locked the car.
4. I once did a home visit to a lady who had recently been discharged from the Maternity Hospital, checked her over, asked the usual questions and commented on how well the baby looked and then left. When I got back to the surgery, I suddenly realised that I had been to the wrong house!!

I should have been two houses further down the road. I found it hard to believe that despite being at the wrong address, I had found a lady who had given birth a few days earlier.

What were the chances of that?? The lady that I should have seen was not really known to me having been seen throughout her pregnancy by one of my partners who was away on holiday, hence me not realising I was attending a different lady. The following day I visited the correct lady at the correct address then popped along to the wrong lady's house to apologise and find out who was her GP. I rang him to tell him what happened, and he was quite happy about it and asked if he could claim the post-natal visit fee for my visit!! Of course, I said, "Yes."

5. I once did a home visit at 3AM and when I went back to my car, I found that the battery was flat, and it wouldn't start. Luckily, the patient's family were still at the door and realised my problem. Fortunately, they had a set of jump leads and brought their car up to the front of mine but when I opened my bonnet, I could not find the battery!! Turned out that the battery was in the boot so after a bit of manoeuvring we got my car going and I got back home. This really showed one of the joys of General Practice. There I was, potentially stranded in the "rough" end of town, but I just *knew* that I would be OK because this family were on hand. I had known the family, three generations of them, for many years and together we had been through quite a few medical problems together. I knew for certain that if there had been no jump leads available that they would have happily driven me home and looked after my car until I could retrieve it later; the type of incident that probably doesn't happen in other branches of medicine.

6. I did a home visit one Christmas Day evening to a man who was having "severe abdominal pain." I was there fairly quickly and on entering the house I found a man sitting at the table having a meal, so I asked him, "Where is the patient? Is he upstairs?" "Oh, no," he said, "I am the patient."

I looked at him again and then down to the meal he was eating. It was the biggest plate of greasy chips, covered in mounds of tomato sauce, I had ever seen in my life and he was really tucking into them. Besides the plate was a large glass of beer and two, as yet, unopened bottles. I was very tempted to tip the whole plate over his head but potential dealings with the MDU came to mind and common sense took over. I took a history, then examined him and, as you can guess, I found nothing amiss.

I let him know, in no uncertain terms, that home visits were for people who were seriously ill and not for people that could wolf down quadruple portions of chips with beer, but I suspect that I may as well have been talking to the wall.

7. I was asked to visit a lady in her 60s (I was going to call her an old lady but then remembered how old the members of the Year of 68 are now) who lived alone and was the sister of one of the ex-partners in my own practice. Arriving at a sizeable, detached house in a nice part of town, I knocked on the door and gently pushed it open as I always did on home visits. However, it would not open fully, and I had to squeeze through, only to find some boxes and a bucket were blocking it. There was an inner door and again it would not open fully although it was not as tight a squeeze as the outer door. Walking through into the lounge and could barely believe my eyes.

The room was full to the brim with items such as excessive furniture, boxes, and the thing I noticed mostly, multiple piles of old newspapers and magazines on every surface, including the floor. Not a square inch (or should it be square centimetre now) of empty space. The newspapers had obviously been there a long time as most of them were now faded and yellow. There were also multiple dirty plates and cups scattered about. There was a narrow walkway through the junk across to the chair on which she sat and another path to another chair on which sat a female relative who had come along to give her moral support.

I thought, perhaps, that she was a bit gaga but no, she was completely lucid and spoke really well with great precision. Obviously a well-educated lady. After taking a history it became clear that I would need to examine her, so the three of us headed along another narrow pathway towards the bedroom.

This turned out to be exactly the same as the lounge, complete with old magazines, yellow newspapers and other sundry clutter everywhere. On the way through the relative kept catching my eye and raising hers to the ceiling, clearly embarrassed about the whole thing. At the end of the visit the relative accompanied me to the door and I asked her if it was worth getting Social Services involved. "Oh, no," she said, "she wouldn't allow them through the door. She has been like this all her life and won't change now. It's just the way she is." Yes, that was the way she was: who are we to say what's right or wrong, or even what's normal or abnormal.

I believe that there is a TV programme about hoarders. She would have been an ideal candidate.

Needles and Pins

Always a great believer in trying to find ways of treating patients without stuffing potentially poisonous chemicals down their throats, in the middle part of my career I took up acupuncture and hypnosis and used them in my practice. I had some successes with hypnosis (a girl with bright red hair who was a trapeze artist and had an insect phobia comes to mind) but had to abandon it after a relatively short time as it was just far too time consuming in General Practice. However, I did keep the acupuncture going as I could put the patient in my side room, insert the needles and then go back to see the next regular patient in my consulting room. After that patient was seen, it was back to the side room to twiddle the needles and then on to the next regular patient. So, the patient having the acupuncture would be in the side room for about 30 - 40 minutes with two or three twiddles of the needles which was just right. For certain problems it worked quite well, muscular neck and shoulder pain particularly. For smoking I had a success rate of less than 50%. I always considered my greatest success was a patient who had suffered with Phantom Limb Pain for over 10 years; after six sessions it disappeared and never returned over the next 15 years that I knew him. It got him off the codeine based analgesics that he had been on which meant that we were both happy.

One day I put a chap in the side room, put the needles in, went back later for the twiddling and then ……. completely forgot about him. After seeing my last regular patient, I noticed that I had finished for the day, left the surgery and drove straight home.

Just after getting home I had a call from the surgery telling me that Mr. H was still in the side room with several needles in his shoulder and neck. Most of my staff were extremely needle averse but, fortunately, the one who wasn't, a nurse, volunteered to take the needles out as long as I agreed. Of course, I agreed and told her what to do if there was any bleeding, as I didn't fancy driving back.

Mr. H took it all in good humour and every time I saw him afterwards, we had a good laugh about it. And his shoulder/neck pain cleared too.

Coincidence? Or Something Else?

We have done quite a bit of travelling over the years and it's amazing how often we find ourselves chatting to, or eating out with, other medics (I include dentists in this group too). You might argue that it is more likely that this group will take similar holidays because they are similar people (similar to me, not very likely) and, presumably, have a similar income. I can understand that and, maybe, this is part of the reason, but it seems to me that there is more than that. I'm not sure what percentage of the general population are medics, but it must be quite tiny.

Once, on a four day rail journey, we were chatting with a couple from Germany who spoke excellent English. We sat with them at a table for four and our choice of table had been quite random. As time went by it became clear that the man and me were both in the medical profession and we both said, at exactly the same time, "you must be a doctor."

He was a GP in what used to be East Germany and remembered well the miseries of Communism. They told us about a recent holiday that they had in South Africa and how much they had enjoyed it. They had stayed in a hotel about three or four miles out of the centre of Cape Town at Sea Point and it looked out over the ocean. Between the hotel and the sea was a green strip and it was here that the paragliders, who had jumped off the mountain behind, landed every day.

Before they could tell us the name of the hotel, we told *them*, "it's Winchester Mansions," a place that we have used a lot over the years and the only place where the paragliders land. They were duly astonished, as were we, at the coincidence.

On another occasion we met yet another German GP and his wife in Kalk Bay, about 20 miles outside Cape Town, and spent a whole evening chatting with them. We were the only four guests at this small hotel that night.

Another time we were in a group of about twenty, and ourselves and three other American couples decided to wander down the street to a recommended restaurant. We barely knew each other, and it was a spur of the moment decision. As we sat eating it became clear that I was not the only medic at the table; one of the men was a Neurosurgeon and another was an Anaesthetist (or Anaesthiologist as he called himself).

A few days after we moved to our present address we were invited to a party by neighbours and there we met a dentist who lived just round the corner. He had qualified in Newcastle in 1969. We became great friends, going on holiday together a few times, and our wives became bosom buddies too for many, many years.
On yet another holiday, after a couple of days with a group of about 16 or 18 people we arranged to have a meal out with a friendly couple. He turned out to be a dentist.
On the first night of a cruise, we went to take part in a quiz and tables of six were needed. We didn't know a soul, but two New Zealanders called us over and asked if we would like to join them, as, "we looked like people who could do quizzes." I'd like to think that we had on our intellectual faces, but I think that they were just desperate to form a team and were buttering us up, so we joined them anyway. A few minutes later they hailed another random, passing couple who also joined the team. Yes, you guessed it, he was a GP from the Midlands.
And then there was the doctor that features in the "Dreaming of Tomorrow" anecdote. And, another time, the doctor who had been in the RAF doing Aviation Medicine. And the one we met in the Drakensberg Mountains, miles from anywhere.
There have been other similar occasions over the years where, seemingly by pure chance, we have met up with medical people, but at our present age it is not always easy to recall every time this happened.
It's not that we got chatting to these people because we knew they were doctors but the very opposite – we found that they were doctors after the chats began. And, of course, we met many folks who were not doctors but I just feel that the number of medical contacts seems so disproportional that it cannot be coincidence alone. What the hell it is, I really have no idea. I'm certainly not a believer in fate, astrology, fortune telling, tarot cards or any other mumbo jumbo (although witchcraft is another matter, as I'm sure I'm married to one). I can only conclude that maybe I have discovered some new fundamental force of Nature – Medical Magnetism.

A Long Way Back

It is a long way to Auckland, New Zealand. But at least we broke the journey by having a couple of nights in Singapore. In Auckland, on arrival, we went to our hotel and wandered out onto the balcony of our room to admire the view. Immediately adjacent to our balcony was the balcony of the next room and a couple of people appeared so we started chatting.

You know the routine, "Where are you from?", "England", "So are we. Which part?", "North", "Where?", "Yorkshire", "Which bit?", "North Yorkshire", Whereabouts?", "Teesside", "Oh, we're from Teesside too, where exactly do you live?", "We live in Acklam,", "Don't believe it, we live in Nunthorpe!"

"Travel the World, meet other cultures, experience different ways of life, communicate with other folks," is the mantra, but here we are, 12,000 miles from home, on the opposite side of the planet, talking to some people who live 3 miles from where we live.

After a bit more general chat the lady looks me in the eye and asks, "Did you used to work at Hemlington Hospital?" "Well, yes, I did," I reply. "Thought so. You were the houseman when I was a nurse on Dr Graham's ward." I was astonished. But I have to say that I did not recognise her or even remember her, but she obviously remembered me. She also knew the names of other members of staff there and that we had one of only three flexible gastroscopes in the UK at that time. And all this was 50 years earlier!! 1968 to 2018.

A couple of years before this incident I had been standing at the bar of our local pub when a chap came up and said to me, "You used to work at Hemlington Hospital."

On this occasion it was a statement, not a question. He told me that he had worked in the labs there and remembered me as the houseman on one of the wards. Being a very small hospital, I found it easier to go into the labs, which I passed regularly, to get info and, also, it was good to get to know the people in there as info extraction was much easier if you knew the staff. Shame to say it but I honestly couldn't remember him. Maybe he had changed.

These two incidents were, in one way, quite reassuring. I could not remember people from way back and I could remember what I did yesterday.

It certainly boosted my confidence, and I was very grateful that it wasn't the other way round. So, two people recognising me from many years back means that there are three possibilities here. 1. As a junior houseman I looked really old, or 2. Now that I am old, I must look incredibly young, or even 3. My appearance is so unusual or weird that people never forget. I know which of the three I would like to think was correct, but Kathy assures me that when I was a houseman, I looked about 12 and that now, at my present age, I have less hair, it's a different colour and that I most certainly do not look young in any sense of the word. She tells me that my appearance isn't particularly gruesome or bizarre, for which I am very pleased, and that people remember me because of my blue eyes. And there I was thinking that it was my rugged, film star, good looks and sparkling personality.
She tells me that I'm nuts.

Dreaming of Tomorrow

Away on holiday somewhere, we got chatting to a couple from the Middle East and were quite surprised at the prodigious amount of gin and tonics they were getting through. Surely against their religion but, then again, no-one's perfect. After a while the conversation somehow got round to dreams. He told me that he had had a recurring dream over many years and that it had started after his five years at University. Well, the five years was a bit of a giveaway and, sure enough, it turned out that he had studied Medicine. He went on to tell me about his dream and it turned out to be EXACTLY the same as one that I had for a long period too.
In my dream it was the evening before our Finals Exam, and I had done no revision whatsoever. On a table in front of me were my entire collection of textbooks and reams of handwritten lecture notes. I stood looking at them thinking, "I've got to read, ***and learn***, all this material tonight before I go to bed." Clearly an impossibility. And that was it, dream ended. I never found out what happened the following day and I never considered the dream as a nightmare. The dreams only began ***after*** that final exam.
I had this dream perhaps three or four times a year for about 20 years after qualifying but then it gradually became less frequent and finally disappeared completely. Maybe I'd finally come to terms with the fact that I had actually passed the exam.

The Joys of Communism

Part way home on a long haul we stopped off in Havana for a two night stay. Always had a hankering to see this once splendid city, now, sadly, mostly run down. We were taken to a smart, modern hotel at the Marina, clearly only for tourists. This was in 1999 when US- Cuban relations were very poor and US citizens were banned. Well, that was the theory but in reality, almost all the boats in the Marina were American and all the surrounding bars and restaurants were full of Americans too. Seems that the authorities, keen to get US dollars, always looked the other way. What's the old saying, "In theory, there is no difference between theory and practice; in practice, there is."

A couple of hundred yards along the street was a clinic and occasionally I would see people going in and out. I can't resist places like this and am always keen to see how things are in other countries, so I wandered along one afternoon and inside found a decent size waiting room with no-one in it. A nurse appeared and I managed to make it clear to her that I would like to see the doctor. She waved me to follow her and took me through to a smaller room where there were two doctors who, fortunately, spoke very good English.

We had quite a long chat about their health system and ours and, although both systems were free at the point of consultation, patients there had to pay the full price for any medication. That was, of course, if the medication was available there at all and quite often it wasn't.

They explained that they were so short of basic medicines, dressings and equipment that the service they provided was absolutely minimalistic. They were even short of writing paper, pens, paper clips and all the things that we never even think about. I must have been there for about 40 minutes and in all this time not a single patient arrived for a consultation. I guess if there's nothing much on offer then there's not much point in turning up. I went back to our hotel.

For many years, when we went on holiday, I used to take a bagful of medical stuff, mainly because we went to some remote third world places. I always had broad spectrum antibiotics, painkillers, antihistamines, Dioralyte, Imodium, plasters, bandages, Micropore tape, needles, syringes and even a small suturing kit just in case the worst happened.

Our own mobile pharmacy. We were flying home the following day, so I picked up this bag of gear, some ballpoint pens, some hotel notepads and marched straight back to the clinic. In the doctors' room, I emptied the bag onto a table, and they looked at me as though I was mad, wondering what I was doing. I said that I was donating all this equipment to the clinic for free. To me it was just a small amount but to them it was huge. They were overwhelmed and called the nurse through and when they explained to her what was going on, she broke into tears. They were very happy, and it certainly made me feel happy too. We've always found that, in general, wherever we have been in the world, the people have been wonderful, it's just the politics (and religion) that spoil everything.

Naivety and Serendipity

I remember so well the day we stood in the entrance area of the old Medical School, someone stood on a box and read out the names of those that had "completed" the Finals Exam (not passed) and we all felt so relieved and joyous. We even received an envelope with the title of "Doctor" on it. Wonderful.

A few days later, Kathy and I returned to sunny Teesside to meet our families. We had actually married in 1967 (no, not for that reason, our first born didn't arrive until 1970) and she had helped support me for the final year.

One day someone asked me what I was doing next and it suddenly hit me - I'd never once thought about getting a job. How naïve could I be? It must have been all that euphoria that clouded my brain. I was qualified but unemployed and unable to support a wife or a future mortgage. Not coming from a medical background, I had no-one to advise or guide me and I simply never considered looking out for a job at my last student post at the hospital.

In a slight state of panic, I rang the main hospitals in the area and the Hospital Secretaries of all of them told me that there were no posts available. I should have applied earlier. I then tried the middle sized hospitals and got the same answer. Fearing that I would be attending the Dole Office each week I finally rang the Hospital Secretary of Hemlington Hospital, a tiny, isolated place several miles out of town. "Yes," he said, "there was a vacancy, and could I start in three days' time?" Accommodation would be available in a few weeks.

The hospital had originally been built during WW1 and consisted of a main corridor with half a dozen spurs off each side.

Most of the spurs were made of wood, the exceptions being the labs and the operating suites which were more modern, brick built and more than adequate. The main corridor actually ran uphill with quite an incline and all the porters that worked there had huge leg and arm muscles from pushing trolleys up the corridor and one worn shoe from slowing the trolleys when going downhill. We eventually got our accommodation, and it was a detached wooden hut with a corrugated tin roof. You can imagine the racket when it rained. Right next to our luxurious hut was a small brick building with a huge lock on the door and outside of which were usually multiple bunches of flowers. Yes, it was the hospital mortuary. Kathy often asked what it was but, because she was rather squeamish about such things, I told her it was the "flower shop" and didn't tell her the truth till years later.

So, I started as JHO in the Surgical Team. How different from the teaching hospitals it was. No ward rounds with the consultant and his huge entourage, it was just consultant, registrar, SHO and me. The registrar was a chap in his fifties who still had the title of Dr. (not Mr.). Seems that he had tried, and failed, to get his FRCS many times but blew it every time when faced by examiners. He was a superb surgeon and could deal with any emergency thrown at him but just couldn't do exams. He remained a registrar till he retired.

Six months on, I moved across to the Medical Ward and once again it was consultant, registrar of a sort, SHO and me. Talk about thrown in at the deep end, but I felt as though I learned a tremendous amount in both of these posts.

The registrar here was actually a GP who had an FRCP to his name and his job consisted of turning up on Thursday lunchtime, having a pretty good free lunch, doing a very casual ward round and then disappearing till the following Thursday. If you can remember 1968-9 then you would know that having a gastroscopy, in those days, was something to be avoided at all costs because rigid gastroscopes were just about impossible to get down. But, at that time, there were three of the new-fangled, made in Japan, flexible gastroscopes in the UK, two of them in London Teaching Hospitals and the third one, believe it or not, in Hemlington Hospital. How Dr Frank Graham got hold of one I will never know but there it was in this tiny outpost and we could actually see peptic ulcers and neoplasms rather than just about make them out on a blurry barium meal X ray. He had referrals from all over the north of England.

I used to chat to the GP with the FRCP on Thursday lunchtimes and he told me that one of his partners had died several months earlier and they could not get a replacement. In General Practice, it seems that there are periods when new recruits are almost impossible to find and other times when they are coming out of the woodwork. He asked me if I might be interested in the position and, having always fancied doing general practice, I said yes, thinking it might be a temporary measure. We decided that I should do a spell in Obstetrics, as that would be needed in general practice, so I went off to do that for six months and had less sleep than at any other time in my life!

So, the big day arrived in February 1970 when I started as a GP. This was before GP training courses were widely available and, as before, it was straight in at the deep end. It turned out that the GP I originally met, because of his FRCP, had a considerable number of local hospital consultants and families as patients and, with large numbers of working class patients, there was a huge range in this practice.

The senior partner in the practice was a really nice, easy going chap and we all got on very well. It was a few years later that I discovered that he had an Olympic gold medal. He had been born in India, his own father, from Northern Ireland, having been in the British Army there. He had been superb at all sports and eventually made it into the Indian hockey team that won gold at the Berlin Olympics in 1936. He was very modest about it, but I did eventually get to see the medal, the only one I've ever seen.

I'd always vowed that I would not return to Teesside to have a career but, of course, once there, and with a wife, two kids, a mortgage and a large Old English sheepdog to support, the years rolled by and I became a permanent attachment. Only once did I consider moving elsewhere and I looked at a job as a GP in Cape Town, but our two daughters were just at the wrong age to go through a major upheaval, so I stayed.

By 2003 I'd really had enough of all the bureaucracy and form filling and retired as a GP. I took up a part time job working for the Offshore Oil Industry, mostly in Teesside and occasionally in Aberdeen, and finished that in 2015. So, I worked for 47 years - I must have enjoyed some of it.

Unusual Cases

1. A Real Rarity

A lady in her early sixties came back from holiday saying that she seemed to have put on a lot of weight around her middle. So much so that she could only get into elasticated items of clothing. When examined she clearly had ascites and I arranged an urgent referral, fearing the worst.

Quite by chance, several years earlier she had volunteered to take part in an Ovarian Cancer study and had been found to have borderline levels of the marker CA 125, known to be raised in most cases of Ovarian Carcinoma. Because of this she had been monitored more closely than most in the trial, but the marker levels remained no more than borderline throughout. She was due to have some further, more detailed, investigations after her holiday but events overtook her.

Paracentesis drew off a large volume of fluid, some of which went off to the lab. It was expected that the diagnosis would be Carcinoma of the Ovary, but Pathology reported that this was Primary Peritoneal Carcinoma. This, too, is associated with raised levels of CA 125 but because of its rarity barely gets a mention.

Chemotherapy resulted in a brief remission and repeated paracentesis kept the fluid down but, sadly, her overall survival was less than six months. PPC is listed as being very rare with only about six cases per million individuals and, certainly, none of my colleagues, mostly GPs, had ever seen a case and in some cases never heard of the diagnosis. It was the only case I ever saw.

2. Cannonballs

A man aged 49 came in and I didn't recognise him; he was one of those patients who had been on the books for years but had never been ill. He said that he felt that his breathing was more difficult than previously, especially if he exerted a little. He was a non-smoker and was not coughing. When I examined him, I found nothing unusual except that his breath sounds seemed somewhat diminished. There were no localising signs and, this being a long time back, we had no Peak Flow or other respiratory gadgets to play with.

I sent him off for X ray and the report was quite stunning – huge round masses in both lungs and a small pleural effusion on one side. I had him into the Respiratory Unit very quickly.

There, fluid was drained from the effusion and the lab report showed the presence of Malignant Melanoma. He was then searched head to toe and a small, slightly unusual "mole" was found on his foot. Biopsy of this also showed Malignant Melanoma, so it was removed. Following his foot surgery, he was sent home with the most horrendous prognosis – a few weeks at most. However, he seemed to pick up and feel better and eventually started to get out and about. He had been given a follow up appointment by the hospital but I'm sure that they never expected to see him. He went along and the X ray was basically the same although the effusion seemed to have gone.

He then attended another follow up, and then another and the X ray always looked the same: huge Cannonball secondaries in both lungs, but no bigger. After several months he even went back to work and the follow ups continued with no change. He eventually began to lead an almost normal life although any exertion made him slightly breathless. This went on for the next ***thirteen years*** with his X ray remaining exactly the same – huge round masses in both lungs but no bigger than the original X ray. He seemed to have developed some sort of symbiotic relationship with his Melanoma metastases. The hospital had never seen anything like it.

Then, one day, he came to see me, and I could see that there was a change in him. He had lost weight and looked grey and gaunt. Suspecting the worst, I got him down to the hospital and this time his X ray had changed – the huge secondaries had become even bigger. It seemed that, for some reason, the symbiosis had come to an end and the Melanoma had taken over. And this time he never even got out of the hospital before the end came, very rapidly.

Tattoos and Piercings

1. He was the most awkward, annoying, and obnoxious patient on our books. I'm sure you all had one, the one you most hated to have to see. Tattooed all around his neck he had a dotted line and the words "Cut Here".

I have to say that I was sorely tempted.

2. She was a young lady in her early twenties, and she had a tattoo as follows "NO ENTRY ↓" It was placed about half an inch above her pubes!! I thought it was a bit OTT but then I considered that anyone going into a Tattoo Parlour and asking for *that, there,* must have had a lot of guts.

3. I'd heard of "having a Prince Albert" but was never really sure that it was a genuine procedure or whether it was just an urban myth. Then one day, there was one before my very eyes as I examined a patient. He was new to the practice so I didn't know him well enough to ask questions, much as though I would have liked to. My mind quickly went through all the possible downsides – going for a pee, other intimate activities and lastly the thought of it catching on something and being ripped off. Advantages, I could think of none. Several years later I saw another one whilst doing a medical. Just thinking about it still makes me cringe. There is no evidence of Prince Albert himself ever sporting one of these. One day, however, someone actually had the thought, "Wonder what it would be like to have a metal ring through the end of my ……"
4. I once saw a lady who had a decorative stud in one of her labia. I couldn't help thinking that if she had one on the other side it could have acted like a press stud – good for closing things up! Ideal for the lady, above, with the tattoo.

Hard Cases

One We had all sorts of patients in my practice, from medical consultants to criminals and hookers (although on thinking about it those groups were not necessarily different).

One day I saw a new patient to the practice, aged 41, and I didn't like the look of him when he entered. He looked and sounded menacing, and I suspected that he might be trouble.

He got straight to the point: he wanted something doing about his face, which was very red and covered in multiple pustules especially on his forehead and cheeks.

His tone of voice suggested that I had better make some improvement to his looks or I might have mine rearranged.

I went through a few questions and he had had acne as a teenager, but it cleared by his early twenties and his present problem had begun in his early thirties and had come and gone over the years but was particularly bad at the moment. It looked like a typical case of Rosacea. I mentioned that alcohol could exacerbate the condition, but I could see immediately that he had no intention of cutting down on his beer consumption.

At that time the simplest and cheapest treatment was oral tetracycline and I felt that simplicity was definitely the best way to go with this character. So, I prescribed Oxytetracycline 250mg daily, which had worked pretty well with other cases, and asked him to come back in four weeks, having explained that there was no quick answer here.

When he returned, he looked a fair bit better, and I noticed that he was not quite as aggressive or menacing. I think he even managed a smile. Another four weeks later there was more improvement and, as each month passed, his face began to look very respectable – not quite like a baby's bottom but a great improvement on the original. Also, he said that his girlfriend was very pleased. And so was I, as I felt much more relaxed in his presence. He became very chatty, and it was almost as if we had become best friends after about six months.

Then, in one consultation, when he seemed very happy, and after a few jokes, he said to me,

"You know, Doc, if ever I can help you in any way just let me know. If ever you want anyone taking out, I can do it for you." And he was absolutely serious. I think that I knew what he meant by "taking someone out" but I didn't know what to say, just nodded and moved the conversation along.

A couple of months later he told me that he was leaving the area and so he left the practice. By this time, I still hadn't thought of anyone I wanted "taking out" although I did flirt with the names of a couple of awkward patients. What a friendship we had made!

Two. I had seen him occasionally with the usual minor childhood illnesses but had no contact with him for a long, long time and could only remember him as a kid. He was now in his twenties and when he came in, I thought, "Wow, you've grown." He was about 6 foot 5 inches tall, had the stature of a brick built convenience and looked very strong. His father had been a professional footballer in the lower leagues and was a really nice chap, but his son had a reputation in the area as a hard nut, often involved in fights and it was rumoured that he, perhaps, ran some sort of protection racket, supplying alarm systems to lots of small businesses.

He had caught his hand on something and broken the skin, but I didn't think it needed stitches.

I suggested that he might have a Tetanus top up. "No, no," he said, "I hate needles." I could see by the state of his teeth that he was not a regular attendee at the dentist. I tried again to persuade him to have the Tetanus jab, but he was adamant that he would not have it.
He went on to tell me that he was absolutely terrified of needles and would do anything to avoid them. I could see in his face that this very conversation was making him shaky. It seemed strange that this great hulk, who was immensely strong, hard as nails and obviously scared the living daylights out of his competitors and customers, was so frightened of a little needle.
I later remembered that I, too, was needle phobic for many years. When I was 5 or 6 years of age, I got measles and, of course, being a future medic, I got the complications. Not only acute otitis media but acute mastoiditis, too, which made me very ill. The treatment, then, consisted of IM penicillin twice a day for ten days: I used to look out for the arrival of the District Nurse, morning and evening, and when she appeared at the door I would run and hide, either under the bed or in the cupboard under the stairs. At that age the syringe looked enormous, and the needle looked incredibly long. I had to be captured from my hiding place and held down as the injection was administered to my backside. It was no wonder that I was scared of needles. I did not look forward to my polio jab several years later but being amongst my school friends, I couldn't be seen to be scared and took it with clenched teeth. I have no problems with needles now.
So, our giant of a man never did have his Tetanus top up, but I always felt that if ever I got into a situation where he threatened me I could simply pull out a needle and syringe and he would run a mile.

Getting Nowhere

When the Covid 19 pandemic began in early 2020 I received an email telling me that my name would be restored to the Medical Register in case the NHS became overrun, and would I be happy to be called up if necessary. I was very happy to agree to this but over the next few months heard nothing more. As the summer progressed the number of cases and deaths fell quite markedly but then when winter came along the numbers rose sharply again and a further lockdown was introduced. But still, I heard nothing.

Then, of course, the cavalry appeared on the horizon. Three vaccines were approved and there was a need for millions of them to be given as quickly as possible. I looked into becoming a vaccinator. There were articles in the papers about non-medics, St. John's Ambulance, firemen etc., being trained up to give jabs in 3-4 hours so I thought this would be a piece of cake for retired medics like myself, having given hundreds, if not thousands, over the years. Then I read a letter in the newspaper from an ex-GP who had applied but had been asked to upload 21 documents before being considered. I thought this was maybe an exaggeration until I looked more deeply into it.

Yes, we were expected to have undertaken various e-learning courses, taken tests and generated certificates in subjects such as Preventing Radicalisation (did I have to check patients' political and religious views before jabbing them?), Child Sexual Exploitation for Volunteers (there would be no children coming to vaccination clinics), Fluids and Nutrition for Volunteers (surely, just eat and drink plenty whilst doing the jabbing), Fire Safety for Volunteers (run out of the building if fire broke out?) plus many other seemingly irrelevant courses.

I didn't think I could manage all this guff but then my daughter, who works for the NHS and has had to do all these courses, despite not having any contact with the public at all, gave me some "assistance" and I ploughed on through the list, took the tests and generated the certificates. This took just over two weeks (3-4 hours for non-medics? Should have applied as a non-medic) so I then uploaded all that I had and, yes, there were 21 documents in all. I got a "Thank You" email in reply and was told I would hear more shortly.

I imagined myself at some local clinic, eating and drinking wisely, wearing my trainers in case I smelled smoke and doing the jabs, feeling that I was, at last, making some contribution. Then I got another email from the NHS. One of the last questions on one of the forms had been "Have you given any vaccinations in the last 12 months?" and I truthfully answered "No." Big mistake: I should have lied and answered "Yes" because my truthful answer has resulted in me being asked to take another three e-courses, take another three e-tests and generate another three certificates.

Anger and frustration. My foot was within half an inch of going through my computer screen when I read it. After three weeks of all this I now feel that I do not have the will to continue. In fact, I barely have the will to live. The NHS seems determined to prevent me from doing something that I have been doing since pre- qualification days: giving IM injections.

I have often read about the fact that over-regulation and red tape cause endless delay and inefficiency and now I have seen it, first-hand, in all its glory. I think that I now have some idea what NHS bureaucrats do all day. They dream up new, ridiculous regulations to justify their very existence.

I am now sitting at home thinking of how many jabs I ***could*** have given by now.

Jeanne Jackson

A few thoughts prompted by the present Covid crisis when thousands of retired doctors have found it very difficult to apply to be helpful because of the need to supply evidence of having attended the many required courses.

My experience has been so different!! I decided to do Medicine when I was 13 ... the French teacher asked us all what we would like to be. I surprised myself and the class so had to stick to it!

My first job was in Surgery at the Ingham Infirmary, in my hometown, South Shields, following a phone call from one of the consultants. My aunt was a well-known local GP and I never knew if she had helped. The cosy doctors dining and sitting rooms fostered quite a family atmosphere. Hugh and I married in December 68 ...we visited the ward in our finery and gave my bouquet to the young girl who was about to have major surgery, then returned to our guests!

After Christmas Hugh returned to Germany to his Army base, and I was offered my next house-job in Medicine in Gateshead, Hugh's hometown. Life was very busy with often overcrowded wards, and we used to cover for each other's departments, so made easy friendships.

In the meantime, Hugh consulted a Colonel in Germany, who commanded the Field Ambulance in Munster, wondering if he had any Civilian Medical Practitioner jobs for me from July 69. The colonel thought I would be too inexperienced, then asked, 'which Medical School?' and his attitude changed to delight...."that's mine too! When can she start?"

So it was that every morning at 7.30 a very smart Scots Guardsman would salute me while standing by a mini...my transport to the Barracks Medical Centre and to families in their married quarters. I soon learnt all sorts of soldierly tricks to get an "excused boots" note for no good reason, and that Colonels of Guards regiments expect wives always to prioritise their husband's Army duties.

Back to England... to an Army base surrounded by little villages, awaiting a married quarter. We had a drink in a lovely pub, chatting to the landlady.

"You can rent our cottage for a few months and the doctor in the next village is looking for help"!!

I learnt a lot about a rural population, "it's the cottage after the 3rd barley field after...", helping in the dispensary, avoiding herds of cows on the roads, and trying not to get the mini snowed in.
The GP was a farmer's wife... they went away on holiday once leaving me in charge. The patients were no trouble but early one morning the pigman was throwing stones at the 16th century farmhouse window shouting,
“Ring the vet...the pigs are eating each other's tails!!"
Many house moves later, in Warwickshire and then to Surrey, several part time GP jobs came my way. Then in 1973 with our 3rd child on her way, Hugh left the regular army, and we came North to be close to our families. We found ourselves living next to a 'year of 68' classmate...he knows who he is!!
Thanks for passing on those locum surgeries when you had other unexpected priorities! I was offered several more part-time opportunities in Blyth which required me to be on call at night, including some police work.
Then, with an ever growing family I was surprised and relieved to be offered a day job in Child Health...no more night calls in those days without mobile phones and with a car that disliked cold weather!!!
There is much more to tell, but in all this time the only proper formal application and interview I remember having was for my last job, in Community Child Health, and that opened up a lot of interesting and varied opportunities over the 21years until I retired.

Dr Kek Foo LIM

Medicine in Malaya

I am a Malaysian Chinese but had the privilege of being a foreigner admitted to the University of Newcastle upon Tyne. At that time, I was the only foreign student from Malaysia / Singapore or Hong Kong, so it was a great privilege.

I came back to work in a tropical multiracial society, mainly Malays, Chinese, Indians and other ethnic minorities. I worked initially in the University Hospital Kuala Lumpur in 1969, as a surgical house officer and the Medical officer in General Medicine. I joined the first batch of medical students in the university. All of us had to work very hard and most qualified as specialists, who worked in Singapore and many became famous.

I stayed on and joined a group of General Practitioners with several clinics. The said practice happened to have a lot of patients with sexually transmitted diseases as some of its doctors were good at treating those diseases. This motivated me to go back to London to pursue a Diploma in Venereology in 1980. It was around this time that consultants reported that young men especially were getting pneumocystis pneumonia and skin cancers Kaposi's sarcoma, cancer in the neurological system, as a result of human immunodeficiency. After much contact tracing, they found that it occurred in homosexuals and sex workers and their casual contacts (the beginning of HIV transmissions).

In my practice in Kuala Lumpur, I had a number of mainly female sex workers who were brought by pimps for medical check-ups. I also later worked with Institute of Medical Research (IMR) as well as Virologists from University Hospital, mainly doing trials, swab samples and blood samples.

I detected the first HIV positive case in Malaysia – a 21-year-old Lao-tian girl who looked quite normal and pretty. At the time, confirmatory testing was done in Australia and the result reported, but the relevant enforcements officers did not do so. Foreign prostitutes who are detained are usually sent back to their countries of origin. In her case, she was picked up by her pimp who decided to take her back to Laos through Thailand. Since then, HIV has been rampant, especially in Thailand. Awareness in Malaysia increased greatly following an incident involving a famous singer.

After all these years, a vaccine has not been developed for HIV. Most other sexually transmitted diseases do not provide immunity, and one can get gonorrhea several times, and syphilis again and again. It is the Papilloma viruses which cause cervical cancer. Viruses do mutate, and in this Covid-19 pandemic, will we be able to develop a vaccine as mutants are already here?
Medicine in Malaysia, as in the world over, will need to be practiced with compassion as there are a lot more poor rather than affluent people around. I have treated blind patients without fees, as they often are brought by their young children to the clinic. One may have to give them the transport fare to come back for follow up visit. Also, in Malaysia, there are a lot of customs / superstitions like whether certain foods are too "cold" or "heaty" and using herbs will enhance the treatment. Frontliners like us must face sadness and tears, sometimes from infidelity, as treatment of spouses or contacts often involve the diagnosis of their situations.

Dag Kremer

Here are a couple of good memories from likely the most important, happy and memorable time of my life.

A case of some unusual balls

First year for most students starting Medical School. (Some of us - about 5 students - had to do Pre-med, that included Physics, Chemistry, Biology) for one year. We were doing Physiology and a course in human metabolism and nutrition that included all kind of measurements like weight, fat, muscle mass, urine output and some lab values.

On Friday afternoon 3 or 4 “volunteers” were picked for the weekend to measure their input in the form of food, fluids and output of urine (no stools) and body weight two-times a day.

It was on Sunday afternoon that my troubles started. We were not to go out to eat or drink. it was getting late, and shops were closed. For my evening meal I only had a tin of Reindeer meatballs called Joika. They were in a can with a picture of a smiling boy and his Reindeer. It was quite popular for Norwegian students to take these cans with us, I suppose to remind us of home.

Monday came; I brought my measurements that included all the weights of what we had been eating and drinking. Plus, my blue empty can of meatballs with the same smiling boy and the picture of the Reindeer.

We were given food tables issued by the War Office. I remember they had a military green cover and contained all the sorts of food you could imagine. I presume for possible war situations from anywhere in the world. But no Reindeer meatballs! There were Swedish meatballs (you know like the ones you get at IKEA), but I refused to use them as that would not have been right. After an extended discussion we finally compromised on some English balls. I was often asked ‘Any Reindeer meatballs lately?’ after that.

“Useful information”: JOIKA or JOIKE is the sing/song to call the reindeers, - like a kind of yodelling. PS: You can still buy these Joika balls, and when I see them, they still make me smile thinking of that amusing day.

Henry

My introduction to clinical medicine, apart from "junior clerk" on the ward, included sitting in with the consultants in Outpatient department. We were usually about 4 of us in the room at a time.

I remember very well the first day in Neurology with Professor Henry Miller. From the start he was in exceptionally good spirits and trying to wake us up and speak back to him.

"You all look depressed", he suddenly said. "For example, him", pointing at me. "Where are you from?" "I'm from Norway". "Oh my God", or something like that, - "and you lot say all the depressions come from Britain".

This was in fact true as the weather report in Norway all seemed to start with - "a new depression is forming over England and coming over here". It made us all laugh and we always enjoyed his stimulating and fun clinic.

A couple of years later I was fortunate enough to be a guide for a visit to Norway of British professors and teachers from medical schools where Norwegians traditionally had studied. They were from Aberdeen, Glasgow, and Newcastle. Wives were included. It was a thank you trip, but also to discuss medical education and politics. We sailed from Tyne commission quay on the M/S Braemar, and it was a most stimulating week full of laughs and fun. They made a great impression on Norwegians and fostered friendship.

The man in charge though was of course Henry M. I will never forget when on the first day he had an hour's lecture in the Department of Health, - everybody was there. He picked up a piece of chalk and said: "There are two kinds of lecturers; those that come with slides and those that come with ideas. I have no slides".

Then he held the audience spellbound for almost an hour with no notes. Unforgettable, -have to admit I was proud. That was the week that was, for me.!!!

Neil Longridge

Chr—t he's stopped breathing.

As an otolaryngologist in Vancouver over the last 40 and more years I have had the experience of several unusual cases. As I see it as a surgeon, anyone who has not had some bad results and made a few errors, which are of course inevitable, then they have not operated much.

Rather than describe my less than successful situations I thought I would I entitle this present epistle "Chr—t he's stopped breathing." Despite working in North America for 40 years I still use religious rather than fecal/ sexual epithets.

The first time I came across a critical airway situation I was moonlighting in the emergency at Newcastle General Hospital while working as a demonstrator in the anatomy department, just after finishing my house year. I had done a little bit of work in the RVI emergency as a houseman, sewing cut fingers and sending off people with acute abdomens to the surgeons. It seemed no different to go and do this for a bit of extra cash at Newcastle General. I had done a few sessions there and invited one or two of my medical students that I was teaching to join me to learn to sew fingers etc. About 11 o'clock one night a child was brought in who had been involved in a fire and had significant burns. He had about a 30% body burn situation and I was just starting to address how to manage this, the medical students having cut off his clothes, when he stopped breathing and I said the inimitable words.

"Ch—t he's stopped breathing."

Firstly, I squirted some intravenous hydrocortisone into his lungs to calm them as I realised they were not working, presumably due to smoke inhalation.

At this point I said, "Get me an endotracheal tube" and by a fluke, as I didn't know how difficult it can be to intubate urgently, managed it first time. Greatly impressing the students to whom the whole process was new, as it was to me. I had never intubated any one since my 2 weeks in undergrad anaesthesia.

Afterwards, he was taken off to the nascent ICU at Newcastle General. I followed him over the next month and miraculously he recovered. The body burns were extensive but superficial, fortunately.

That was my first episode of "Ch—-t he's stopped breathing" however over the years I've had a number of others which I will briefly recount.

The second event of this sort occurred after I had been working at the RVI in the ear nose and throat department for about three days. Although I was inexperienced, fortunately I had spent six months running the Newcastle General Hospital ICU as Alf Petty's registrar and had experience of tracheostomies. Under my care we admitted a patient overnight with a large fluctuant lump in his neck. In the little room under the stairs to the doctors residence at the RVI we were sitting discussing the lump in his neck before the days' surgery began. I said that if I had seen this man in the emergency at NGH I would have drained the abscess in his neck (which was either a very large lymph node or a brachial cleft cyst.) At this point my colleagues interest perked up. Hugh Marshall went and checked him out and agreed it was probably a good idea to drain this abscess immediately. The process was set in the motion and I got the honour of doing the procedure as I had suggested it. The anaesthetist did his usual induction with curare, paralyzing the patient, but unfortunately due to neck swelling was unable to intubate so it wasn't quite, "Ch—-t he's stopped breathing."

But still very worrying, though we were scrubbed and ready to go. I then proceeded to do my standard tracheostomy with Dick Watson the SR as my assistant and to his credit he didn't take over. It went well and rapidly which after three days working in the unit greatly impressed everyone. Because of the quick procedure we completed our whole list early, with me as an observer as I knew no ENT operations.

A month later I was called by the staff at Gateshead General Hospital in Low Fell where I would be observing Jeffrey Chaytor examine patients. I was not able to assess a patient properly yet and I was just in the training process.

It was the custom at that time that you did not call the consultant for an emergency and I as registrar with only four and a half weeks experience was called instead. It was 2am, I drove across the Tyne bridge to the hospital which I had been to only twice before, checked the patient and decided to operate.

I had to find out where to change and at the exact moment I walked into the operating suite the patient stopped breathing. It was an 18-month-old child with acute epiglottitis, and this really was a

"Ch—- she's stopped breathing."

So, with no scrub and no gloves I did a very rapid tracheostomy on this tiny infant. Probably more by good luck than skill I opened the airway without much bleeding or any other damage and inserted the smallest endotracheal tube the hospital had. The benefit of this urgent type of procedure is that it is fast, clean, and over quickly, which meant that only 20 minutes after reaching the hospital I was back in my car and going home with the child being taken care of by an anaesthetist. As I recall, sometime later he was the unfortunate man who fell asleep and died on his way home having worked for 24 hours.

The third of these events occurred after I had been in practice in Vancouver as an otolaryngologist for about 15 years, still needing to be on call and maintain my familiarity with tracheostomy. I was called in to check out a patient in the middle of the night. Vancouver is different to the England, it is expected and insisted upon that the surgeon in charge is in the room when the procedure is done. Therefore, I had to get up and go in, as this this man was having difficulty breathing. I was in the emergency department looking at this individual lying, obviously very distressed and short of breath, when suddenly he sat up at 45°, pointed to his throat, and collapsed unable to breathe. Fortunately, in the emergency room there is a tracheostomy set.

On this occasion gloves were available which I quickly put on, AIDS had come to town, and proceeded to do a very rapid tracheostomy with instant breath restoration. This was a very rare situation, he had acute adult epiglottitis. The main benefit once again of having an acute event like this is that it is rapidly dealt with, rather than having to arrange for the patient to go up to the OR where a great deal of the jockeying would take place to get access to the 1 or 2 overnight operating rooms. I was on my way home 20 minutes after I arrived, just like at Gateshead Hospital.

This was much better than the previous week when, in the middle of the night, I had to deal with in a man who had laryngeal Ca and stridor who turned up in extremis with acute airway obstruction. It was obvious we had to get him to the Operating Suite as fast as possible.

There is a huge vulnerability between the emergency room and the operating suite. I called in advance to say,

"This patient has an acute airway we are coming now."

Giving them a chance to organize in advance and we set off. I rushed as fast as I could, pushing the stretcher with the nurse. She was quite small and angrily questioning why I was rushing so much. It is two floors, an elevator ride, and then a long corridor, during which if an acute airway crisis happened it would be virtually impossible to do anything. This was the reason I was rushing. She was complaining vociferously about me all the way.

Tracheostomy is a very standard routine procedure except it wasn't this time. The man was desperately short of breath and I did not feel it was safe to have the patient intubated. So, under local anaesthetic, I did a transverse incision and found that the trachea was moving up and down approximately 2 inches with each breath. The patient was very short of breath, so it was very rapid movement, making it very much a difficult moving target. At last, I managed to get him to hold his breath for a moment and plunged the knife in, at which point he took a huge breath, relaxed, allowing us to complete the procedure, and he went off to the ward. The whole event took somewhat under 40 minutes before I was on my way back home. The night nurse took me aside after I finished the procedure and said she had talked to the emergency nurse who had complained angrily about me because she was very upset that I had been so rude to her and what right had I to do so as a hospital porter! I guess I was wearing thrown on clothes. Once she found out that I was the surgeon she decided she would not make a formal complaint.

Not all tracheostomy's have a happy ending. When I was Alf Petty's registrar at Newcastle General, I was requested to do a tracheostomy on a patient on whom I'd assisted with a cancer of the stomach removal the week before.

Halfway through the procedure the bleeding stopped abruptly, and the anaesthetist informed me that the heart had stopped, which wasn't really so surprising as the patient was really in very poor health. Although a very unpleasant outcome for me there was a small benefit, the head nurse of the unit took me aside and gave me a cup of tea and a biscuit and became much more friendly than she had been to me for the rest of my time in the job. She was widely known as a somewhat tough lady, so although the result wasn't good for the patient it wasn't all bad.

A few more thoughts.

In my left shoulder, as all people my age do, I have a scar representing vaccinia damage due to smallpox vaccination. Well done Jenner. The word is vaccination for Covid being used in BC is incorrect and immunization should be used. This was the first substantial medical development of modern times, modern being over 200 years ago. Subsequent to this many descriptions of diseases were made. Addison, Bright and Graves the great man of Guys described their diseases about1850.

Ménière, in my field of otolaryngology described his disease at about the same time and the cause of this is still unknown. It was not until the 1920s that much in the way of treatment occurred. I was fortunate in being George Feggetter's last houseman, 1969. For those of us who remember him, his main round was on Sunday morning, his main outpatient session was on Saturday morning. This was because of the 9/11 system as he had an extremely large private surgical practice. In 1969 with a flu like illness known as Hong Kong flu was the pandemic of the time.

I did get it and worked with fever and some rigors, no doubt passing it round. As a houseman you didn't take time off. For me it was a relative bonus as all the surgical beds were closed except for emergency surgery for a period of about a month. This was also the time of the beginning of ICU. I recall an anaesthetist Jo Stodart having a 16-year-old girl die of acute collapse from this flu and breaking into tears. The patient was dehydrated had a gradually increasing pulse and then suddenly there was a catastrophic blood pressure drop. It was this patient that resulted in the local ICU developing a treatment of pouring in saline and Ringers fluid when the blood pressure disappeared, and no subsequent lives were lost.

I recall Mr Feggetter specifically describing to us during Sunday morning rounds that as a houseman himself in 1923 he was sworn to secrecy because at the Edinburgh royal infirmary they had discovered that feeding patients with raw liver on dry toast cured pernicious anemia and planned to present it at the RSM and didn't want the news out before the presentation. For those not aware of medical history 1923 was the year insulin was discovered and this was really the start of the mushrooming explosion of medical knowledge that has gone on since that time.

Harry Jones a general surgeon from Sunderland, who sadly died of hepatitis B, described working as senior registrar to Mr. Feggetter some years previously. Mr. Feggetter said, 'I'm on call this weekend call me if you need me here's my phone number, deal with any emergencies that you can.' The phone number was a club in Pall Mall.

Another Mr Feggetter story was that Napoleon had been winning the battle of Waterloo and unfortunately due to severe pain from his piles caused by riding his horse he had to go and lay down in his tent during which time the battle was lost.

In my time the development of CT scanning and MRI meant that it was possible to precisely define the size and extent of skull base tumors. With a neurosurgical colleague in Vancouver, I was fortunate to be able to develop local expertise in this field. Patients were easily available as previously they were untreatable. Necessarily this type of surgery being completely new was done extremely slowly and cautiously. It was essential to read up the anatomy in the days prior to surgery and in fact go to the postmortem room and anatomy department to undertake direct dissection in people who no longer had concern about this. Following this we undertook a series of procedures, largely successful with relatively little harm done, where we restored relatively normal functional appearance in previously majorly handicapped people. As I've said this was slow sometimes requiring a reference to textbooks even in the theatre. One particularly uplifting occurrence was when having started the procedure at 8 AM one morning we had been alternating bouts of 2-3 hours each and as we were starting the closure the morning staff came back on duty the following day. Fortunately, this was an only occurrence but does indicate the duration and type of effort necessary to accomplish these complex procedures.

I was registrar in general surgery working with Mr. Petty and Mr Dudfield Rose at NGH, he enjoyed and was good at cholecystectomy. This required me as his assistant to retract the spleen and bowels for him to get at the area. Mr. Rose was bald and like Bobby Charlton and Donald Trump curled a long piece of hair from the back across the skin at the front.

While leaning forward from the patient's right side in order to see the anatomical area of the gallbladder this lock of hair, as he did not wear a hat, flopped down and at the end of the procedure not in frequently was coated with blood. A politically positive decision on my part was not to inform him of this although I'm sure he noticed it in the in the changing area afterwards. I gather it had been difficult to persuade him to start wearing gloves many years before. Nobody had convinced him that a hat was indicated. He was a very kind man and invited the medical staff and nurses to his home, a small castle up the coast with a sea view and an amazing antique collection.

We tend to forget that surgeons in the UK are called Mr. because they arose as a separate group from physicians and apothecaries, they were barbers. The reason for this is that the barber is the man who sees people with infective disease due to bad teeth and bad teeth was a major cause of death due to airway complications in the 19 century, so dealing with neck abscesses became their skill and so were Mr surgeons born.

We also don't appreciate that in the 19th century syphilis was common. Approximately a third of the population in Victorian England had syphilis. With respect to this John Kilborn in the year I joined 69, became a star when recognizing a patient with recurrent pyrexia of unknown origin in a patient at St. Mary's mental hospital Stannington. She had tertiary syphilis, he suggested that they do a blood smear looking for malaria as induction of high pyrexia was a method used to kill treponema pre antibiotics, it was positive. I only saw one patient int the UK with syphilis in the neurology ward at NGH, with Tabes Dorsalis acquired from a Mademoiselle from Armentieres in Flanders. I have seen from northern B.C. one secondary syphilis with sudden unilateral sensorineural hearing loss and 6 bilateral progressive hearing loss tertiary cases in First Nations people, due to either infection acquired sexually years before when young or congenital, probably carried to them in the pre antibiotic time by Caucasian fur trappers who were a rough and ready group.

Ursula Martell

Complications of contraception.

This incident happened more than 40 years ago but the look of dismay on my small boy's face is with me still. It was the reception class turn at the school assembly and my boy had the main part. We had practised over and over and at last, he had done it, I could relax as all I had to do now was keep the baby on my knee quiet for another few minutes. Then the headmistress announced that she wished the children to listen to a special radio broadcast the following week.

I started to fish in my bag for my diary to make the appropriate note. My bag of course was full of nappies, wipes, toys, assorted bric-a-brac and an IUCD (intra uterine contraceptive device) in its loading device. At that time new IUCDs were being produced at an astonishing frequency all very much the same, all a little different. I used to carry the latest edition with me so I could familiarise myself with the one handed technique at any opportune moment.

As I picked out my diary, I must have hit the button on the device as suddenly the little horror was catapulted out, it flew up in the air at an amazing speed, performed somersaults over the heads of the children and finally landed at the feet of the headmistress. There was a sudden silence and I remember hoping that the headmistress, an elderly spinster, would think it was some sort of toy.

This was not to be, Dave Harle who had been in the year ahead of us and was then a local GP was sitting next to me, He announced clearly and for all to hear that it was no surprise I had 4 children since I kept my coil in my handbag!!

Mike Marshall

A Miscellany

It was in my first or second week of my house job at Shotley Bridge hospital, when I was duty doc in A&E on a very quiet Sunday afternoon. A lady limped into my consulting room with an ankle bandaged. As I bent forwards to look at the injury, I noted the bandaging was virtually useless and hanging off. When I asked her what had happened she said "it's not my ankle doctor. I've just pretended it is the problem, so I don't have to tell my husband what's wrong" I was intrigued by that point, but I was flabbergasted when she revealed all! " I have a condom left inside and I can't get it out" So I replied in all innocence "why couldn't you say to your husband?" She replied "'cos it wasn't him who left it there". This was the beginning of my postgraduate education.

The next incident was when I was surgical registrar in Sunderland General hospital. I was on call when I had a phone call from sister in Sunderland Orthopaedic & Accident Hospital late one evening. She described meeting a man with " a vibrating tool up his anus". It just so happened I had recently looked at an article concerning practical jokes in the workplace using compressed air tools, and how dangerous they can be. I asked how the chap was and sister said he doesn't seem in any pain but is very nervous. I asked her to arrange an abdominal Xray and I would be there within 15 minutes.

After I arrived, I waited for the patient to return from Xray. When I saw the Xray all was clear! He had a vibrator in his rectum and nothing at all visible at his anus. I asked for a sigmoidoscope and a set of Cheatle forceps and set to work to recover the device. We did manage to get it out by pulling gently on the vibrator with the forceps aided by the patient bearing down. All he said to me during the procedure was something like "don't grip the bottom end and twist it at the same time or it'll start up again" No damage done but he was a bit sheepish when I left.

I learned later he was presented with a box containing the vibrator by the nursing staff, who had tied a bow around it.

As a general practitioner from 1979 I worked in family planning clinics for Durham and later Sunderland Health Authority. One night I did a locum session in Chester-Le-Street clinic. One of the ladies I was to see was requesting a smear.

When she was advised I was the doctor who would do it, she asked if I was married. If I was, I could do it, but if I wasn't married, I couldn't do it. I was and I did it. Another incident involving a smear occurred in my practice in South Shields, where I took a smear from one of our patients. As I turned to put the specimen in a plastic bag, I said something like " everything looks healthy there" and she replied, " so it should be it's hardly ever used".
Another lady patient in South Shields was a frequent attender as she had restless legs which at that time didn't have any particularly effective treatment. She attended several times over a few months, and I wasn't making much progress easing her problem. One particular day she said to me " I don't know, doctor. I think I should have this leg off and get a wood one. What do you think doctor?" I said to her "I wouldn't bother - knowing you you'd probably get woodworm in it" She burst out laughing and I never saw her again for several months, but we remained friends.
One evening, after a busy day in South Shields surgery I had yet another "extra" to see at the end of surgery. This young chap said, "I feel as if I might be sick". I said, "have you been sick?" He said "no - but I feel as though I'm going to get pain in my belly" I said have you had belly ache?" and he said "No". So, I examined his chest and abdomen after taking his temperature (normal), after which I said, "I feel as if I should find something wrong with you, but I can't".
He then left, seemingly reassured and I never saw him again!
Early in my GP career in Durham I had seen a 14-15 yr. old lad with his mother in afternoon surgery. I cannot recall his immediate problem except he had pain which had not responded to paracetamol, or Solpadine (in those days!). He had been nauseous and so I prescribed a couple of naproxen suppositories for a trial. Just before I left the evening surgery, his mother called to say he was in agony and she thought it was due to the suppository. When I called and examined him, it was the suppository, except it hadn't been removed from its plastic covering, which says a lot about his determination.
I had a particular patient who often seemed excessively anxious about health matters, even though I never saw him for any serious illness.

On this occasion he was needing some analgesic for his arthritis; as we discussed his options he suddenly piped up and said "I divvun want any o' them "penicilliums" 'cos ah'm illogical to penicillium, and ah divvun ' give us them "distelastics" (Distalgesic) or "cocobanas" (co-codamol). It was hard to keep a straight face sometimes.

I used to attend post-grad lunches/lectures at James Cook Univ Hospital, and one event was a lecture from either an MDU or MPS representative, who touched on the question of what abbreviations had often been used by doctors in patient records: most I had heard before, like GOK ("God only knows"), FLK ("funny-looking kid"). The best one, which was new to me, was a good one - TFBNYD. This meant "totally fucked but not yet dead". Such entries were of course entirely unacceptable and could result in legal action if ever discovered.

My final years in general practice were in Teesside, In February 1992 I joined a longstanding private practice based in Bridge Road, Stockton on Tees. The senior doctor was David Redman, who had prior to joining the practice had been intending to become a hospital physician. This practice evolved from the surgical practice of Watson Alcock in 1793. Over the years there had been some notable names associated with the practice, including Dr Hodgkin of Redcar and "Towards Early Diagnosis" fame, and apparently Henry Miller who ultimately became Professor of Neurology in Newcastle.

I was appointed to replace a prominent partner about to retire, namely Aubrey Colling, who had been very much involved in the development of general practice of vocational training in Newcastle. Aubrey had been co-author of a paper in 1976 suggesting that certain heart attack patients might be safely managed at home rather than in hospital.

I thought he was an excellent doctor, who was extremely popular with his patients. Beyond that he was an excellent musician, who studied composition at York University after he retired. He looked after sheep and kept bees at his home in East Rounton, North Yorkshire. During the second world war he trained as a pilot in the RAF, but I am unsure as to whether he saw active service.

The practice had its own pharmacy which was an important source of practice income.

I invited a good friend of mine, a pharmacy lecturer at Sunderland University, to review the pharmacy and he was impressed with the cost effectiveness of the drug range on our shelves at that time. I left the practice after three years, mainly because the salary increase, I expected never materialised, so I returned to NHS practice, initially joining our colleague Pete Irvin in his North Ormesby practice, and then on to re-forming the North Ormesby Health Centre practice, where I worked until 2006, when I retired from full-time practice.
In 2003 Meg and I moved out to Weardale to live in a farmhouse between Stanhope and Eastgate. Although it was in so many ways a beautiful place to live, going to work took on a new dimension, given that Meg worked at North Tees Hospital, and I worked in North Ormesby, so we each had a 40+ mile commute each way.
We normally travelled separately, and usually I left home before 7.00am to avoid heavy traffic around Teesside. Sometimes Meg and I would arrange that I pick her up at North Tees, and we travelled home together. One morning after travelling home together the previous evening, I set off for work as usual. It was only when I was passing Wynyard - possibly 35miles from home - I realised I'd left Meg behind. I had to dash back, to find Meg about to call a taxi. Suffice to say we got back to Teesside in reasonable time, but I lost a lot of brownie points that day.
On another morning driving in I felt a strong cold draught on my feet, again probably around Wynyard. I quick feel around confirmed I still had my slippers on! I must have looked very relaxed to patients and staff on that day!
Together, these incidents perhaps were telling me life was getting a "bit too much" with all this hectic commuting. So, there you have it. The digression about the Stockton practice, was to put into context the pressures we had going to and from work, leading to my senior moments above.

John Milne

Interviews

In my junior hospital days, I became familiar with most regions of England. I travelled far and wide attending interviews for which my reticent nature was unsuited. Four interviews are memorable.

The first took place in a London teaching hospital for which there were several applicants. After the interview we awaited the result which was the usual practice. The minutes passed, thirty, sixty, one hundred and twenty. We thought it must be a difficult decision and we all became anxious and restless. The boyfriend of one of the competitors came looking for her. He was not as patient as us. After a further twenty minutes he suddenly stood up announced he wasn't going to wait any longer, strode angrily across the room, flung open the door, with our hearts in our mouths we watched in admiration, only to find the interview room empty. It was a very impressive performance. Needless to say, he worked in financial circles. The interviewers had omitted to tell us that we would informed of the result by mail. What a bovine lot we were.

On another occasion I had received no response to my application. At 6.30pm. one evening whilst working late in the cardiac department of UCH the phone rang. A voice at the other end asked who I was, followed by well are you coming to the interview, they are underway. I explained that I hadn't received notice of the interview, and left immediately, realizing the possibility of a positive outcome otherwise they wouldn't have called. The interview was a success, and I accepted the post. On taking up the job I learned that the head of Human Resources, a lady of forceful personality, had considerable influence over some consultants and was capable of manipulating outcomes. She obviously had someone else in mind for the post.

The most memorable and disappointing non interview followed an application for a consultant post. The senior physician of the hospital phoned to invite me to a pre-Christmas lunch with the other applicants.

On my arrival the embarrassed host took me aside to inform me that the full appointments committee had not shortlisted me, but I could stay for lunch. This was an offer I found easy to refuse. It turned out the committee had been encouraged to appoint a time expired registrar they were having difficulty placing.

His appointment was not an altogether success. Interestingly he was a colleague of mine. The fourth interview of interest was another of my many failures. One of my referees was a Freemason who had contacts at this particular hospital, and he was very encouraging. Unfortunately, days before the interview he put a dampener on my enthusiasm. A Freemason had applied for the job which scuppered my chances.

Fortunately, all worked out well in long run and I had many happy productive years in West Essex. The overall message is that interviews are not always as they seem nor as they should be.

Allan Myers

Memories of Domiciliary Visiting

In late summer 1978 I moved to Blackburn Lancashire from Hampstead North London, taking up the post of Consultant Cardiologist and General Physician. On my first day at work, I discovered the “joys” of Domiciliary Visits. At the time unbeknown to me these requests were commonplace. The GP would contact my secretary requesting a home visit in time honoured fashion. A note would be left on my desk with the patients address and clinical details. I was expected to visit the same day.

Being well before the time of sat navs and mobile phones, I would have to find my way to the patients home using a flimsy A to Z and the light of a torch, even when I was to meet the GP at the home. I was initially unfamiliar with both the narrow hilly terraced streets and the high rise blocks I encountered. Such visits were generally in the evening following on from the usual working day. Most often it appeared to me that these home visits took place on dark, wet cold typical Lancashire evenings.

On just such a night I found my way to a little terraced house, upon knocking at the door, I was aware of barking dogs. The patient who lived alone took some time to answer the door then took me into his back room. I was aware of two very large dogs in the backyard leaping up and down at the window. Having ensured that they were secured I proceeded to examine the patient. He had bilateral infected varicose ulcers embedded with dog hairs and wriggling maggots among other things. It was clear that admission was necessary. I remained with him whilst he arranged for dog care. During the wait for an ambulance, I talked to him about my dog, a relatively small cocker spaniel.

I next met him two days later on the ward round, a typical nightingale ward of 24 beds, his ulcers had been cleaned by this time and the infection had settled and he was feeling much improved. The patient was slightly deaf and had a very loud voice. He reminded me of our discussion about dogs, I had explained to him previously that a neighbour wished to mate her female cocker with my small dog but so far, he had not been successful in this endeavour.

The patient in words that could be heard by the whole ward went on to describe in graphic detail methods used to enhance successful mating. This included digging a hole for the larger female to be placed in, allowing my small dog to reach the female relevant part. This was followed by a vivid description of turning the dog during the mating process. At this point I became aware of a deathly hush outside the curtains as the nurses and patients followed the discussion with great interest, culminating in guffaws of laughter from all corners. Needless to say, I was much more successful in my treatment of the patient's legs than I was in arranging the siring of puppies.

Patients present at the time reminded me of the event whenever they attended outpatients and the ward round that day was etched in staff minds becoming a part of the ward folklore.

Some weeks later I was asked to see a lady in a high rise block, I had been informed that the patient was complaining of chest pain. I found the correct tower block eventually after some difficulty. I trudged up eight flights of stairs as the lift was not working carrying my case and my weighty ECG machine.

I knocked at the appropriate door which was answered by a lady who appeared to be expecting me. I asked if she was Mrs **** and she replied that she was. I explained who I was and that I had been sent by the GP. She invited me in. After taking her history and examining her I performed an ECG. The patient clearly had angina. I explained that I would advise the GP on a change to her medication and that she would be seen in outpatients in a months' time.

On arriving home, I called the GP with my conclusions only to hear that his patient had telephoned him to inform him that I had not arrived to see her.

This was a great surprise and concern to me as it dawned on me that I must have examined the wrong patient.

It became obvious that I had called at the wrong address and examined the wrong lady. Subsequent investigations revealed that I had been given the incorrect flat number. I visited the correct patient the following evening and repeated the process of examination, diagnosis and advice after apologising profusely for my nonattendance the previous evening.

The GP followed up with a home visit to the first patient who explained to him that though she realised I should be seeing her neighbour she thought this was too good an opportunity to miss for a specialist consultation.

One cold evening some months later I was asked to see an elderly patient with a history of chest pain in one of Blackburn's more prosperous areas, I found the house without any difficulty, the door was answered by the patient's wife who was expecting me to call. I introduced myself and she told me that her husband was in the front room sleeping and that he seemed much better. She showed me to the room where he was and told me she would leave me to see him on my own.

I entered the large rather cold room, introducing myself to the patient from the doorway, but elicited no response. The patient was sitting facing an unlit electric fire. Moving closer into the room I became somewhat alarmed when I realised, he was unresponsive and clearly had been dead for some time. I examined the patient to confirm death and that resuscitation was not appropriate. I was well used to death in hospital, but this was my first experience of death at home. I then had to think about how to explain the situation to his wife. I suspected that she would ask if I was certain that he was dead so decided to record a limb leads only ECG as proof, if needed.

My ECG machine, however, was second hand which I had bought from the Royal Free Hospital, this machine was temperamental in cold conditions and needed to be warmed up prior to using. This necessitated me switching on the fire before I could continue to record the ECG. I then left the patient sitting as i found him and went to find his wife.

I made my way to the kitchen where his wife was and sympathetically explained that her husband had passed away some time before my arrival. I had confirmed this with an examination and an ECG which I showed to her demonstrating a clear flat line, so indicating that resuscitation was not appropriate.

The patient's wife seemed reassured that his death had been peaceful, and I took her to see him before advising her to call for a friend to come and I waited until they arrived.

This was the only time in my career of domiciliary visiting that I had occasion to record an ECG on a patient that had been dead for some time.

These experiences of domiciliary visiting early in my consultancy helped me to understand the many and varied domestic circumstances of patients and their families living in Blackburn and its surrounding area. Most of which became very familiar to me over the coming years.

This taught me never to underestimate the resilience and resourcefulness of the local population. Blackburn people were similar in many ways to Geordies, straight talking and generous. This was one of the many reasons that despite my long hours and the weather I never regretted my move to Lancashire.

Duncan Newton

Old Memories

Some of my most vivid memories relate back to Student days and even before.

There used to be a scheme whereby various physicians and surgeons would agree to cover North Northumberland and the cottage hospitals at Alnwick and Berwick on Tweed. I was, I think, a final year student with Euan Cameron, a highlander from Inverness who was a brilliant physician at Ashington Hospital. He could have won a medical University challenge.

One day he took me up to Berwick to visit the cottage hospital. We went at lightning speed up the A1 and mercifully pulled off what he clearly regarded as a racetrack, for a brief pit stop at a charming town called Belford.

We entered a modest bungalow where the local GP was waiting to go and see a lady in her 70s who had not been well. I was asked to examine the lady who had fairly obvious signs (mercifully)of a classical right lower lobe pneumonia. When all the medical side had been dealt with, I was encouraged to chat to her. It turned out that she had looked after Beatrice Webb in the late thirties to her death in the early forties.

Beatrice Webb was an extraordinary woman, a co- founder of the Fabian Society, a founder of the New Statesman and also of the London School of Economics (LSE) She asked her research assistant William Beveridge if he would be the first principal of the LSE. Beveridge of course prepared the seminal work to found the National Health Service. So, we chatted to the lady who had a beautiful North Northumbrian voice. I asked how was Beatrice domestically?

"Well," she said, "She was helpless really...she couldn't even boil an egg."

Beatrice had done a tour of the Soviet Union with Sidney her husband and George Bernard Shaw the playwright. Their visit was summarised in a 1000-page document.

"The Soviet Union, a New Civilisation?"

The question mark was removed in the second edition after AJP Taylor had described it as the most preposterous book about modern Russia ever written.

His view was supported by Malcolm Muggeridge who wrote for the Guardian about the millions of deaths in the Ukraine from the Starvation engendered by collective farming. Unfortunately, Gareth Jones, the Times correspondent who had written about the Gulags and the famines could not add his word as he by then had been shot by the NKVD in Manchuria. (If any of this interests you, also look up the diabolical Walter Duranty of the New York Times).

Henry Miller

We used to live about a mile and a half from the sea as the crow flies. Druridge bay was the epicentre of our beach life. I must have been 10 or 12 when a family turned up, their youngest was the same age as my younger sister, who was about 6. I must have been about 10, it turned out he was some sort of medical doctor who covered North Northumberland and furthermore liked it so much that he had bought a weekend house in Belford. His wife was apparently called Eileen and as the man slipped off to have an invigorating swim Eileen began chatting to my mother,

"The problem is we have a lovely weekend and as we drive all the way from Belford to Jesmond on the Sunday evening Henry is dreaming up suggestions for supper."

If the powers that be wished to remove Henry Miller from the clinical scene by allocating him to monthly exile to North Northumberland, it clearly backfired spectacularly. His clinical skill rapidly became legendary and he was apparently rated as one of the finest of physicians before he concentrated on neurology.

I can remember some of his lectures almost verbatim. Word somehow went round the hospital that he was lecturing, and the new lecture theatre was packed, with half the people from years below or on the staff. I was lucky to be allocated to one of his clinics which he was taking, backed up by Graham Teasdale and the Australian John Prineas (who taught me to say "Good Day" if you weren't sure of the precise time around noon) the former becoming famous as a neurosurgeon for the Glasgow Coma Scale and Prineas achieved great eminence as a neurologist.

The next patient had come over to see Henry Miller from Blackpool, about 4 hours' drive at best in those days. She had been held up in traffic and I just had time to read the initial consultation, some 10 years earlier. She had developed some progressive neurological disease with tremor difficult gait etc. and was unable to go to school and basically bed bound.

Miller had examined her and commented that he was not entirely happy with her iris. He sent her across to Dr Howitt who arranged a slit lamp examination and confirmed the presence of Keyser-Fleischer rings. Miller wrote to the GP with the bad news of Wilson's copper storage disease and the absence of treatment.

Two perhaps three years later there was another letter in the notes to the GP in Blackpool.

"Dear Dr... you sent a young girl two or three years ago who turned out to have Wilson's disease. I was talking to a Dr Walsh in Cambridge last week, if she is willing to come back to the Royal Victoria Infirmary in Newcastle, we would like to give the new treatment a go."

At this point the door flew open, a beautiful if flustered young woman entered, hugely apologetic for being late, but seemed to all the world entirely normal.

At crucial times in life, it is lifesaving to have a good clinician.

Newcastle General 1968

When I think back to my early days in medicine, I still reflect with a degree of amazement at how thin the medical staffing was.

The RVI, mentioned above was very much the teaching hospital, rather beautiful in parts, relatively well equipped and staffed and pleasantly situated in the city.

My first job was at the General Hospital, with 3 consultants running a paediatric department. Christine Cooper was the physician I first encountered. She was disliked by the social workers and the nurses as she had trained initially as a nurse and then as a social worker before reading Medicine at Cambridge.

Accordingly, she was then disliked by some of the male doctors, who were perhaps more accurately terrified by her, because she was so smart. I remember one of the neurosurgical consultants leaving the ward a dithering wreck, after he had failed to convince of some planned procedure on a child.

She worked in partnership with Dr Chris Davidson who also had a wonderful brain and would give us impromptu seminars on subjects of our choosing, which were invariably very demanding. You would think he had prepared his talk for a week or more.
On one night the lineup was me (with 3 weeks experience) a night sister and a registrar, Kolum Gupta. Both he and the night sister were marvelous and were vital to keeping the whole show on the road.
On this particular night it was extremely busy, and we were all working flat out. I had diagnosed an acute appendix on I think a 12-year-old, Thomas. I was told to ring Dr Davidson who would come in to confirm the diagnosis. He was on call and full of enthusiasm, despite his advanced years, but he was babysitting as his young wife was having a night out. After speaking to the senior paediatrician I was given authority to ring the Senior Surgeon, a Mr Fegetter who was also covering for the Paediatric surgeon that night. Mr Fegetter had a gentle but Socratic discussion with the young boy and posed the question.
"Would you like an operation?"
The answer came back a very firm "No" Mr Fegetter accepted this, but the ward sister said,
"Dr Newton and I will have a further discussion with Tommy".
In we went to the cubicle and she said" Now listen you little blighter, you have this operation now or you'll have me sitting with you all night". Her language was more explicit, but he changed his mind and was home a few days later after a successful operation. It was invariably the senior nurses who saved the day.
Newcastle became famous for introducing and developing the integrated Medical course. I was always very grateful for the teaching we had at Newcastle. Although it didn't score many points on the C.V. and was tedious at the time; the emphasis on exploring the domestic and social background as taught by the Paediatric departments certainly stood me in good stead. In later life. It also revealed that real life is more interesting than most novels.

Brian Pike

Mistaken Identity

In the early hours of New Year's day when GPs were called Family Doctors and actually did their own night calls, a distressed lady rang me, reporting that her husband had just passed away. He had suffered with heart problems for many years. It was my turn on the Christmas Rota to cover the New Year period. The house was located on one of the local council estates and being New Year's Day people were still out and about and in good humour. As I was about to grab the bag, I saw a rather smartly dressed man walk up the garden path and knock on the door. I assumed it was the local minister, he was quickly ushered in and I decided to give him a couple of minutes thinking he could probably do more for the deceased than I could. I gave him a couple of minutes before proceeding to the door. However just as I was about to knock, the door was flung open and out staggered the same man looking as if he had seen a ghost and muttering "I was only first footing" He disappeared down the path at great speed. The deceased's wife told me she assumed the first footer was me and took him straight to the bedroom to certify death!!

Gone to a Better Place

Our Practice ran a branch surgery in a nearby former mining village. There were no appointments, patients being seen on a first come first served basis. Being the junior in the Practice I did the Monday morning surgery so there was usually a full Waiting Room and a queue forming in the corridor.

It was a particularly difficult surgery with lots of ongoing problems, so it took most of the morning to see everyone. Some of the patients seemed a little tense and were unusually keen to depart as soon as they received their sick note, prescription etc.

The Waiting room was also unusually quiet, and I was about to investigate when a lady blurted out that one of the more senior citizens of the village had fallen asleep in the chair and remained in a deep sleep. Rather than wake her those waiting to be seen had jumped the queue.

A hasty examination confirmed my suspicions. The poor lady was a frequent attender always with minor problems.

I assumed that as she lived alone, she came to the Surgery for a bit of company and a chat with the doctors. She obviously felt safe and warm and amongst people she knew when she passed away. You can imagine how quickly this spread round the village and over the next few weeks my surgeries were much less busy. Fortunately, this all happened well before Harold Shipman came on the scene!

Dem Bones.

"And can you describe the car Sir?" My beloved Morris Minor was no longer outside my digs in Jesmond, where I had parked it the previous night. "Yes Constable" I replied.

"It was sandy beige, reg. OAJ 306, split windscreen, a small dent in the front offside wing, a lot of rust around the door pillars and a femorised gear stick!".

"Could you spell that Sir" he said licking his pencil.

Several months before I had been wondering what to do with my half skeleton. Most of the bones were in poor condition and the skull suggested the deceased had something nasty like syphilis. However, the femur was long and sturdy and fitted beautifully over the gear lever which extended to the floor and the femoral head fitted in to the hand perfectly when changing gear.

The car was found abandoned the next a few streets away. Maybe the thief was too shocked to drive it further.

WA

I was a bit miffed when the Medical Superintendent at Port Hedland hospital in Western Australia, said to me at our first meeting.

“Well, what's wrong with you, mate?"

Liz and I had just spent 6 months driving 18,000miles overland to get there! However, we soon found out that " normal" Australian medics did not venture beyond the city boundaries.

I was standing in for a Scottish Doc who was down at the rehab. centre in Perth drying out. Most of the other medics had various problems - addiction to Pethidine, Turners Syndrome, Achondroplasia etc. Despite their various afflictions they were all very competent Doctors, working in an extremely difficult and hostile environment and were great fun to work with.

Dr Dewar

Dr Hewan Archdale Dewar was the first Cardiologist in the UK to provide a doctor staffed ambulance service for Coronary Thrombosis. This was in the early 60s. He persuaded his staff to participate and he set an example by sleeping in the hospital when on duty. This rota included cover for the CCU which was sited on his ward.

He was probably best known as a pioneer of Fibrinolysis. He was always meticulous in everything he did and expected the same attention to detail from those around him. Consequently, he was held in some awe and trepidation by his juniors though behind that rather formal exterior you could on occasions see a twinkle in the eyes.

On one of his duty nights, he received a call from the CCU. For some reason he took the wrong turning and was seen wandering along one of the corridors by a junior nurse. He was always very smartly dressed even at night. On this occasion he was wearing a nice silk Paisley dressing gown, over neat pyjamas and a matching cravat. The nurse put her arm around his shoulders said.

“Are you lost pet? Let me take you back to your Ward"!

The late Dr Alistair Brewis, respiratory physician, was a good friend to Dr Dewar and gave him much help in his later life. He confirmed that this event took place. But he could not confirm the claimed follow up that Dr Dewar's response was.

“Do you not know I am Dr Dewar?!" to which the Geordie nurse replied

" Aye pet, and Ah'm The Vorgin Mary: now let me get you back to your ward.”

Dr Brewis wrote Dr Dewar's obituary in the D&NMGA Newsletter, stating accurately and not unkindly that "Good cheer was a commodity somewhat rationed by Hewan."

I remember Dr Dewar was very fastidious about his diet. On his nights on call he would have breakfast in the Docs dining room. While we tucked into eggs and bacon etc, he avoided all dairy products. He lived until the grand old age of 96years.

Perhaps we should have followed his advice.

A former GP recalls asking Dr Dewar in 1972 to do a private domiciliary visit in an affluent suburb. At the end of the consultation the patient asked what he owed as the fee. The reply was " Ninety guineas - in cash please".

That is a moustache-bristling £876 in today's money. A registrar at that time was paid less than £40 per week - and paid tax on it.

David Powell

What life was like.

I was a junior houseman and was asked to accompany the consultant on a house visit, lord knows why.

It was to a very run-down area of Wolverhampton. We arrived, knocked on the door, it swung open, the consultant stepped in and disappeared. The floor was missing. The front door was the only one in the house. We eventually found our way to the back room where the family was sitting on boxes around the biggest colour tv I had ever seen.

"Ers upstairs" with a pointed finger, we found our way to the stairs, there were no risers. The patient was lying on a mattress on the floor, an old lady in pretty poor condition.

The Consultant was not going to examine her there so I organised an ambulance, back at the hospital, no phone in the house and of course no mobile.

She was dirty, starved and dehydrated, but recovered well.

Tony Reed

M.B. not so bad B.S. undeserved.

All the best stories start with "It was a dark and stormy night". Well, it was a dark and stormy night in October in the Newcastle General Hospital and I plus the rest of our alphabetically linked cohort we seated in the students' waiting room. It was our first day attached to Surgery and we were wearing our pristine white coats and adorned with our badge of office namely our now vintage stethoscope. The registrar burst into the room in the manner of James Robertson Justice and announced there was to be an appendicectomy. He eyed us all then pointed at me and said, "and you will assist". OMG as they say. After the ritual of scrubbing, gowning and gloving up he handed me a scalpel and said cut from there to there. I think I managed to scratch the first superficial layer of the epidermis much to his chagrin. Well, the line wasn't exactly straight and at the end of it all and after stitching up my mentor said, "well if this chap needs to look for the person who started this operation, he just needs to look for Zorro".

And so it went on. Thank goodness there were openings in General Practice. However, I was not out of the woods because the Practice was really keen on did everything a GP could do. We took on just about almost anything that GP's faced in those days.

At interview I was asked about experience etc. and it was intimated that I needed skill in minor surgery. When I said my nickname was "shaky hands" they laughed but little did they know! So, I bluffed my way for many years and did my share of minor stuff. Some people, the ones I fooled, even thought I was competent. As time rolled on and senior partners retired our younger generation seemed less inclined to take on this minor stuff and so it was left to just two of us to hold the surgical fort.

Then came my comeuppance. I had gained some skill in removing the cysts that occur in the scalp by removing them whole and almost bloodless. Since I did not shave or trim the local hair for the operation all the women were referred to me.

Then came Marjorie who was a 75-year-old semi-retired nurse who worked in the local hospital. Margorie was very prim and proper and when she came to the surgery she was always dressed in her best and had her hair done and her nails polished. Her cyst was about an inch in diameter so nothing out of the ordinary and it came out complete with no problem. After closing the skin there was a persistent bleeder so I asked my practice nurse to pass me the cautery blade. As the element glowed the bleeder stopped but Margorie's hair burst into flames. I blew on it which made it worse while my calm assistant silently soaked a swab and dowsed the fire. All Margorie said was "can I smell fire?" From that day on I made sure that all patients were told not to wear hair lacquer!!

It didn't quite end there because in our practice everyone and that was staff, nurses and doctors met at 10.30am for coffee and a natter and to put the world to rights. When I entered after the fateful event the room was in hysterics. My practice nurse was recounting the tale and at the end told the audience that "after Margorie left and saying how grateful she was I had said, and I quote.

"I didn't know whether to blow on it or piss on it".

A confession.

We have all witnessed irrevocable changes in Medicine during our lifetime none more so than in General Practice. The practice I joined in Cumbria was a mainly rural one based around a market town and we did from before the cradle to the grave care. I had been retired 12 years when this tale unfolded.

I live on the top of a hill about half a mile out of Pooley Bridge. Our minor road is popular with cyclists and those with insufficient gears tend to pull into the side of the road at the entrance to our drive to repay their oxygen debt. I was coming back to our house from the village when I saw 8 cyclists to the side of our drive in a state of recovery. I just gave a wave as I passed and pulled into the carport. One of the cyclists removed her cycling helmet and only then did I realise that this peloton was composed entirely of women as they were all shrouded in Lycra, over-trousers, gloves protective glasses and helmets.

The one who had taken off her helmet first had waved and called my name and I recognised her as Michelle, a former patient. She had looked after our twins when they were small and I had delivered both her children, one of them by forceps. I went over to give her a hug and have a craic and she introduced me to the rest of her group. We asked about our respective families and I struggled to remember names and other details. I am sure you all do the same. Michelle is a bright and buzzy lady and she casually turned to her friends and said "Tony is or was our family's GP. He delivered my kids and seen bits of me even my husband hasn't".

That outburst momentarily stunned the group and after a short silence a tall woman at the back said.

"He has seen mine as well" with a somewhat embarrassed sheepish look that is if sheep have a "look". Other hands were raised along with an unscripted "me too" confession.

It turns out that of the 8 women all were from our Practice and I had delivered or been at the deliveries of 6 of them and it made a total of 14 children.

This presence or actual act of delivering children does not happen now and almost certainly never will again. Now I think that is a shame because the statistics for our 11-bed maternity unit were as good as any and better than some. I mourn its passing. (me too PT ed)

The Liaison

Although I would have liked to have tried single-handed practice this was not to be. I worked my whole life in what was a five man to eventually become a mixed 7-person practice. What held us together for my 35 years were the coffee and tea sessions. Everything ground to a tick-over twice a day. Some of the time was allocating visits but a lot of it was just the craic. In fact, one of my older partners when he left confided in an emotional moment.

"I shall miss some of the patients, but I shall really miss the tea and coffee breaks".

It was during one of these sessions that this story was told.

Elsie is a lady now in her sixties. Married with 2 children both married and living away from home. She is a very slender, some would say scrawny woman with a very large bosom.

Although that is not quite the case since she actually wore a very large brassiere stuffed with old pairs of tights. The tights sort of flew out if one had cause to examine her chest when she had one of her frequent chest infections secondary to smoking 30 cigarettes per day. Elsie obviously felt the need for a more fulfilling relationship away from her overweight, aggressive and rather Neanderthal husband. Elsie found a soulmate in the form of a very short, skinny lorry driver who happened to wear a full blonde toupee. In those days Hoover appliances were made in South Wales and sent all over the country and some went to Glasgow. The drivers swapped trailers in the lorry park in Penrith.

We, the partners, were highly amused at the vision of the two lovers conjoined in the back of the trailer with one holding on to his toupee and the other clutching her bosom trying to maintain some control over the flying tights.

Eventually, as in most cases, the secret got out. Unknown to Elsie, Bert (the cuckold) borrowed a car from a mate and went hunting for the lover. He obtained an address on the outskirts of Cardiff and took off to do serious bodily harm to said lorry driver.

After a 5-hour demanding drive he eventually found the house in question and having had a pint or two to summon up extra courage he banged on the door. Standing before him he found a four foot something wisp of a man who was not blonde but completely bald. Bert said something like "oh sorry wrong house "and set off back to Penrith.

I still see Elsie wandering about town looking a bit forlorn but at least with no visible bruises. She is still with Bert. To be honest I don't remember noting whether her bosom is anything untoward now.

Coping with fear

One would've thought that five years of medical school and three years of vocational training for general practice would've made us fit to cope with just about anything.

I first met Alf when I was 40 and he was about 10 years older. His full name is Alfred Lightfoot, and he was a native of Lincolnshire. When Alf was a child, the family moved out to Zimbabwe and started a lumber business which proved to be very profitable. Sadly, the ruling regime changed after his parents died, he was forced to return to the UK.

He eventually settled in a small cottage in a hamlet 10 miles from our practice premises.
He is a bachelor, and his only companions are two elderly grey parrots (70 and 52 years old) and a small flock of free-range hens.
Alf suffers from severe COPD which is not helped by his inhalation of 20 full strength Capstan every day. He rarely leaves the house now except to feed his hens.
His neighbours usually bring the shopping although I believe he grapples with online ordering now.
This tale begins with a visit I made out of the blue as I was passing his lane end. I hadn't seen Alf for several weeks, so this was an unannounced visit, and I was surprised to see his extremely old Fiat 500 was not on the drive.
I knocked on the door for several minutes and the only response was a knocking sound which was the imitation of the sound I made by the two grey parrots.
It was a fine day, so I just had a wander about his garden and smallholding and spoke to the odd hen. I noticed that between him and his distant neighbour there was now a very significant fence made of very strong pig wire topped by double barbed wire.
This structure was definitely new, and I could not imagine it was any of Alf's doing. Being a nosey b**ger I walked closer and tested it for strength and it was obviously a very professional erection.
The neighbour's property is considerably larger than what Alf has and there are lots of Rhododendrons and large shrubs right up to the boundary fence. Whilst gripping the fence there was a slight rustling noise to my left, I turned my head and there in front of me and two feet from my face was a full-grown Lion complete with mane.
I cannot actually recall whether I sent my trousers to the cleaners!
The background to all this, which I later learned from Alf, is that his neighbour had migrated from the South of England. This chap had invested in a large area of pasture and moor in the valley of Mungrisedale.
His hopes were to start a full-scale wildlife park. He had not done very much research into planning restrictions in the Lake District National Park and his plans were refused with no likelihood of ever being passed. He then resorted to purchasing a property locally as he had already acquired several wild animals with which to stock the park. All his attempts failed, and he gave up the idea.

Alf was quite sad really as having a lion next door made him feel like being back in Zimbabwe. The other neighbours were not so generous as the roaring at night were somewhat disturbing.

Big Geoff

My favourite partner was called Geoff or Big Geoff when not in hearing distance. He was a Newcastle graduate, but it was Dunelm then. He stood 1.9m or 6ft 3ins. in old money.

He was well made but not obese. He was a quietly humorous man with great presence. He had played front row for Medicals, so he was not to be messed with. As an example of his sense of humour he always drove small cars around the practice and at the time of this anecdote he drove a Simca hatchback with a totally inadequate engine. His last working car was an MG Midget. With the roof off the car, he looked as if he was wearing the vehicle. With the roof on there was a significant dome where his head distorted the fabric. Now then cast your mind back to when GP's carried out home visits and even enjoyed them as a way of escaping from the telephone (no mobiles then). Geoff was on call and "it was a dark and stormy night". At 1.00 am he received a request for a home visit for the wife of a farm worker. She had a pain in her chest which had lasted since suppertime and had never experienced anything like it before. He did the usual things… switch on the electric blanket for his return, wake the wife to tell her she was in charge and where he was going. He went downstairs and put on as many layers as the Simca would allow and tried to calm the dogs who thought they were going for "walkies".

The Patricksons were a nice couple who lived 8 miles from where Geoff lived so he was pretty much awake by the time he arrived. The farmhouse was a pain in the neck to get to. It was along a long lane which was unsigned and easy to miss especially in the dark with pouring rain.

There was also the agony of having to get out and open a succession of 3 five bar gates. You had to park in the open field and then unlatch a tricky garden gate all the while holding your torch and diagnostic bag.

Save to say all the indications were Mrs Patrickson had suffered a heart attack. Geoff's first action was to phone for an ambulance and then refer for admission.

Mary was still in some discomfort, so Geoff felt analgesia was indicated so he needed to get his other medical bag from the car. Now I did mention it was a “dark and stormy night”, so he had to fumble in the boot of his hatchback with his torch in his mouth. The next day he took up the story for himself and the rest is in his own words.

“I could hear nothing but the wind howling but then I had the distinct feeling there was someone or something behind me. I could feel the hairs in the back of my neck go up, but I knew I had to look. I slowly turned round in my crouched position and there, a foot from my face was the Patrickson’s pet donkey. I thought I was going to need a second ambulance!”

Gloria

This is all about Gloria. I shall call her that because she is not glorious. She was a patient of my partner when I joined the practice, but she aligned with me when he was on holiday and stuck to me thereafter. Lucky old me!

For those of you who remember the Tellygoons she is the spitting image of Eccles. She is blessed with a face like a metalworker’s bench, not so much a twelve-o clock shadow but a modest beard and a voice reminiscent of the foghorn at Souter lighthouse. She has always worn a sort of “shift” dress in a curious oatmeal colour. She wears open sandals all year round which expose unwashed feet and toenails like a parrot. In later life she carried two elbow crutches, but they were used mainly as a fashion accessory. At all times and in all situations, she addressed all partners and staff by their first name. This is fine by me, but it irritated my partners beyond belief. Everyone avoided her whenever possible especially at the children’s school but later in life I noticed she had other friends of a similar social standing.

She and her partner lived in social housing with 3 children, two girls then 13 and 11 years and a boy who was a toddler of 2 years when I took over the family. Only myself and our brilliant health visitor ever made home visits. Social services and the local police avoided them like the plague or Covid. All home visits were for the children and although she appeared caring she was totally feckless.

In one episode the youngest daughter had D&V and I suggested that Gloria should just try giving her clear fluids and I would call back.

Later in the day when I turned up, Gloria had bought some chips to settle Andrea's nausea. Andrea wasn't touching them but Wayne the toddler was standing next to Andrea's moquette armchair with a dirty nappy round his ankles eating the chips after wiping off the excess grease on the chair arm. The poor child looked unwell, so I arranged admission much against the wishes of the Paediatric department!

After every visit I or my HV would follow things up and the children survived but probably by their own, and by now copious antibodies. Her living conditions (of her own making) were so bad that after many complaints by neighbours she was rehoused for modernisation. The workmen said that this is the worst house they had ever seen and refused to touch it until it had been fumigated! The description of the living conditions could benignly described as Dickensian. Whenever I visited her home Gloria would invariably say "I'm sorry Tony but I haven't had had time to clear up today". The kitchen was bare and by that, I mean devoid of plaster. There was a gas cooker in the middle of the floor connected to the distant wall by a flexible pipe. There were two cabinets devoid of doors and a small fridge of indeterminate age. All the other rooms were littered with discarded clothing, full ash trays and empty beer bottles. Thankfully, I never had cause to go upstairs. However, in the corner of the living room resided the biggest television currently available (albeit seriously soiled)

Roll on 20 years of "care" by me and the children had all left home. Now then, what I found surprising was that after cohabiting with a rather feckless partner for all that time he chose to leave and go and live with his father. Gloria was distraught but what seemed to me amazing was that three days later she had a new partner in situ! Obviously, a man of discriminating taste in partners.

In addition, the Children….

The eldest, is a Solicitor and a County Councilor, another runs a successful Taxi company and almost single-handedly raised enough money to save the local cinema. She is a volunteer for several local charities and the third has his own computer company and lives in East Anglia. None of the children speak to their mother.

22 years ago, after the death of my mother, Gloria offered me horizontal counselling! Before you ask…I declined! It is sixteen years since I retired and when I visit our local town centre I am still frequently greeted with "Hello Tony" at 90 decibels. Isn't life great!

Every day is a school day.

If you are a gardener either by design or "force majeure" and happen to live north of the Wash, then you probably watch Beechgrove Garden produced by BBC Scotland from Aberdeen. If you don't then you should. One of the original but now retired presenters is a wonderful guy called Jim McColl. He is knowledgeable and yet humble and would listen and learn from anyone with an interest in any aspect of gardening. His motto is "every day is a school-day".

It took a while for this motto to sink into my consciousness. I suppose after 5 years of Medical School and three of VT it is fairly common to think you know more about Medicine than the patients, but my patients taught me more about illness and even life itself than I would have ever believed.

This is a tale about Bill. I originally called him Mr Summers, his closest nicest neighbours called him Old Bill and the others Mad Old Bill. Bill lived on his own in an ancient touring caravan in a sandstone quarry. There was a large shed nearby and an earth closet. His water supply was seasonal in that it depended on a stream which dried up in summer.

To say he was isolated is an understatement. Bill was one of two children born in a council house in the nearby village. His father owned the quarry but when his parents died, and his sister moved away he had no option but to move into the quarry as the council refused to allow him to stay on his own in the family home.

So how do I come into the picture. Well, one afternoon there was a call from a gamekeeper to say he had not seen Bill knocking about for a few days and he was concerned. Bill was not our patient apparently nor anyone else's come to that, but he eventually became one.

He answered the door when I knocked but he had no idea who I was of course and very frightened by my presence thinking I was some sort of bailiff or certainly not a friend. It took a while to gain his confidence and several visits of increasing length. Why bother …. well, I was fascinated how someone could subsist and live below the radar for 30 years on his own. During our first chats it seemed obvious to me he had schizophrenia and he was in an awful unkempt state and undernourished.

He wanted no intervention, and his thoughts were very disturbed and controlling. Why not section him? I decided it would probably do him more harm than good and it would definitely destroy any trust I had gained. He agreed to let our local district nurse visit and she eventually persuaded him to have some beneficial injection to boost his appetite and help drive his demons away. The anti-psychotics worked wonders and he admitted to me he could now masturbate well without feeling guilty! I don't think he told our nurse though!

I learnt a lot from (I could call him Bill by now) about life on the edge and how it feels to have debilitating mental illness. He lived without any money. Everything was barter and the currency was sandstone paving slabs. His clients were mainly local and in exchange for a slab or two they brought food, batteries, calor gas, clothing and the odd Men Only magazine.

You can imagine that during the years I looked after Bill there were many funny but interesting experiences. My district nurse came in to see me in some distress with severe back pain and right sided sciatica. Mary does not complain easily, and this was a new experience for her.

She asked if someone could look after Bill for a while at least until her back improved and I couldn't understand why. I asked if he had been making any sexual advances or inappropriate suggestions although I thought it unlikely. No, it's not that she protested it's just that after she had given him his 3-weekly injection, he insisted on paying her with a huge sandstone slab and lifting them in and out of her car was just too much. She told me she had paved most of the garden around her bungalow by now.

After about a year Bill invited me to look around his shed (which was about four times the size of his caravan). I asked him what was in it and he told me it was his sculptures. This sounded fascinating. His whole life Bill had been carving fireplaces out of his own dressed sandstone.

They were magnificent. One of the exhibits was in the shape of a huge guitar standing on its body. The sound hole was where the fire was laid. The neck, finger board and headstock were the chimney breast. The frets and strings were carved into the stone. All of this stood about 10 feet high. Next to all of this structure was a portrait of Segovia who was Bill's hero.

On the main wall was an enormous structure about 10 feet wide and of similar height. Bill called it his interpretation of the universe. The firebox was the sun and coming from it were rays of sunlight carved in the very wide chimney breast. Also carved in relief were numerous stars and the moon in its half form. It was awesome and I commended Bill on his skill. I had really got into it by this stage and around the edge of all this sculpture there were semicircular stones which seemed to set things off. I said to Bill "I suppose these must be cloud formations then". "Of course, not Doc" he replied, "they are women's breasts." Hmmmm.

The last scenario was during the build up to the Queen's Jubilee. Bill had decided to celebrate the occasion. Strung from his caravan to his shed were line upon line of bunting.

When I was invited into his caravan there were cut out portraits and press cuttings of the Queen covering every surface.

On his kitchen table was a sort of Ikebana Japanese decoration with dried flowers, a couple of decorated teaspoons with pictures of the Queen, a small brooch with her majesty on it and a large metal clip.

I said to Bill "I see you're celebrating the Queen's jubilee then".

"How did you guess?" says Bill,

"Oh, you are clever Doc I see you spotted the Jubilee Clip". I accepted the compliment gracefully.

I looked after Bill for 24 years until his peaceful death in his caravan in his sleep. Mary and I were the only ones at his funeral.

I really liked old Bill. He taught me so much about life and how to be at peace with oneself. He had deluded thoughts till the end, but they were harmless and inspirational and immensely creative. I mourned his passing.

The Ultimate Road Traffic Accident

When I joined the practice in Penrith in 1972 it was already heavily involved in prehospital care.

The partners all had cars fitted out with resuscitation kit and a little magnetised flashing green light on the roof. Like Topsy this group grew and grew until when I retired it was then a formal charity and I hung around as a trustee. At one of the meetings two years ago one of the GP's reported an incident to which he was called but thankfully had little in the way of serious injuries to report.

At first we wondered why he was bringing it up because it wasn't even reported in the local newspaper and most things are. This one should have been!
Now read on ….
There is a farm not far from our house just off the main road to Ullswater. The family is called Jenkins and the teenage lad is called David. Now David is not the brightest star in the sky and up this point he had already wrecked a tractor and a car but thankfully with no injury.
This particular spring morning dawns fine and bright and as usual Father Jenkins is allocating the tasks for the day.
"Right David I want you to take the UTV and check on them ewes (pronounced "yows" in Cumbrian) in bottom pasture.
This is a field adjacent to the A592 the main road from Penrith to Ullswater. A UTV is a small farm vehicle which is like a two-seater Quad bike with a cabin and a loading area at the back but not accessible from the cab.
"What am I looking for says David?" Well, just go round them and see they are moving OK and not ready to lamb" says Dad. AND be careful with that UTV you daft bugger.
David trots off with Patch the collie in tow. He does a round of the flock in the UTV with Patch enlivening the sheep to make them trot about. One of the sheep, let us call her Molly but she doesn't answer to anything, is reluctant to get up. David is inspired by his diagnostic ability and decides to take Molly back to the farm to let Dad have a look.
Now at this point David is in a quandary because normally Patch travels in the front of the UTV with David but the truck bit at the back has fairly low sides and Molly who is very nervous at this point would be likely to jump out. Hmmm. So, David puts Molly in the front and Patch in the back.
Fair enough, all is well. When David reaches the gate to the A5902 he has to get out to open it.
Now at this point several things happen.

1. David slams the door of the UTV.
2. Patch barks at a passing car as he always does.
3. Molly gets a bit hysterical and jumps partially off the seat leaving her rear end in the air.

Now it just so happens these UTV's are automatic and one of Molly's hooves landed squarely on the accelerator pedal with the result that the machine takes off at warp 9 along the A592 with David in hot pursuit and Patch barking encouragement. I suspect David was shouting "F" words and "our Dad will kill me".
The first hundred yards went without incident but there is a blind corner at this point and coming the other way unknown to Molly is a tour bus.
Being a popular holiday destination, this coach was bound for Aira force with 53 Japanese visitors on board. The bus driver could not avoid a head on collision. He stopped the bus and got out to check the damage and find out what was going on. David used his mobile to call the emergency services. Meanwhile 53 tourists blocked the road to take photographs of everything including Molly. It was an excited gathering I am told.
Our Emergency doctor had nothing to do. Patch was in shock. David was banned from everything.
Molly well, she has decided not to go for her HGV licence.
No animals were hurt in the telling of this story. I did take photos of the UTV.

Alan Rich

Physiology

Now in the glorious 21st Century even the most Luddite of us Class of '68 have probably subscribed to some part of modern technology; WhatsApp, Zoom, Skype, mobile phones or whatever. But do we remember how basic life was in 1964, the era before techno?
Some of our first year teaching in physiology included practical classes which involved the stimulus of a nerve, and the recording of the response; classically, the isolated frogs leg. The lab technicians, in brown coats, set most of it up for us, but we still had to prepare the recording equipment. This was a clockwork-driven rotating drum. To provide the recording surface a sheet of paper was held over a smoking flame so that the soot deposited reasonably evenly over the paper. The sooty length of paper was wound round the drum. To record the physiological stimulus the clockwork was started and a stylus, stimulated by the experimental conditions, moved up and down to record the results by scraping a line in the soot. Once the experimental run was completed the sooty paper strip was removed and varnished to make it permanent. Only then could the analysis begin. And it took and age to get the soot and varnish off your fingers.
I suspect this scientific recording technique had not changed for several hundred years before 1964. What a difference the next seventy made.

First Time on the Wards

Our first exposure to real life medicine was an attachment to a clinical 'firm'. A firm was two or three consultants who between them looked after sixty or seventy patients. These were usually in beds in two adjacent Nightingale-type wards, male and female. It was very rare for the firm's patients to be bedded outside these two wards. If additional capacity was required, up to twelve extra beds could be put up in the centre of the ward where the firm could easily look after them. 'Safari' ward rounds were unknown.
As medical students we were taught and gained experience by taking histories and examining patients during our attachment. However, we did have some duties. These revolved around the 'side room'. This was usually close to the 'sluice' where bedpans and urinals were stored, emptied, washed and re-cycled.

Clinical protocols required regular testing of urine and faeces. The specimens from the contents of the bed pans were collected by the nursing staff who then transferred them from the sluice in open specimen vases, usually with some glee, to the side room. It was the duty of the medical students to test the specimens and record the results.

Unfortunately, there was no great enthusiasm for doing the tests. Then, these involved near-field physical contact using dip-sticks, and the temporary suspension of the olfactory senses – no automation. So the samples tended to fester away in the sluice. As the summer moved on they became riper and riper and I dare say that many were thrown away and/or their results fabricated. Luckily, no-one ever seemed to audit the results, possibly because audit had not been invented. However, many a romance is rumoured to have its beginnings in the side room as fingers met over a specimen bottle.

Real Responsibility

Our clinical attachments in subsequent years were much more hands-on. We became familiar with the daily paraphernalia of clinical work; drips, syringes, catheters, naso-gastric tubes and the like.

Much of this equipment in the 1960s was re-usable. Syringes were made of glass and came separately wrapped in two parts, the barrel and the plunger. The two were not always a good fit. This, together with the need to open two packets and keep the parts sterile while assembling them, made any task requiring an injection rather prolonged. Hypodermic needles were metal throughout, pre-packed and reusable. Allegedly they were resharpened when they returned to the sterile supplies department, but in reality most of them were pretty blunt. Of course, all this was before the days of AIDS and new-variant CJD.

The apparatus for intravenous drips was similarly crude. The IV fluids were contained in glass bottles with rubber caps. A large needle on one end of the drip tubing was used to puncture the bung. It was not unusual to see a little disc of red rubber floating around the bottle. The drip tubing was also red rubber and there was little or no flow control, only a off-or-on gate clip. No drip pumps. In the sixties the presence of particulate matter in the bottles was not recognised, so there was no filter in the drip line. Presumably most recipients got a dose of glass and rubber particles with the intended fluid.

In the House

During our first year as a real doctor (albeit with provisional registration) residence in hospital was compulsory. This is perhaps not quite as bad as it seems as there was no charge and rooms were usually serviced by a housekeeper. My room in the RVI overlooked Leazes Park Lake so it was not unpleasant, although I did not get much of a chance to view it. There was a waitress-service dining room solely for the use of the house staff and the nursing sisters. Elsewhere in the Infirmary there was a Registrars Dining Room and a canteen for everyone else. The lasses(!) waiting on us looked after us well and would always find something if we turned up late for a meal. Meals were free, although sometimes the quality was so poor it would have been an insult to charge for them. I remember calling down the catering manager because there some worms squirming in my fried fish. He said he would investigate and went off to check the kitchen. A few minutes later he returned to tell me he had inspected the fish bin and "only a few of the fish in the bin had worms." At that time NHS premises were exempt from food hygiene regulations. Our salary was £125/year, and my first take-home pay was £5 by the time tax and my GMC registration fee had been deducted. The fee was supposedly a life-time fee, but the GMC seemed to have lost that concept over the following 50 years!

My first job was with Dr Dewar's firm, a physician specialising in heart disease. Work had just been completed on a four-cubicle coronary care unit at the end of his ward, 14. It opened the day I started, and the house officer was expected to sleep in a bedroom on the ward. Unfortunately, there had been no planning on how the unit would be staffed. As a result, I spent the first three weeks of my career sleeping (or not) in a makeshift doctor's bedroom on the ward without ever getting a chance to visit my room in the doctor's residence to unpack my suitcase.

In those days the RVI had a private ward, Pavilion Three. The ward had its own chef and kitchen, and patients were permitted to order alcohol. There were pre-printed private prescriptions which listed gin, whisky, sherry and champagne. House staff were expected to assist with patient care, and it gave me great pleasure of an evening to journey along to the ward, do a round, and write out prescriptions for champagne.

House officers weren't allowed to staff the Accident Room but were expected to attend there to work up emergency admissions to their ward. There were two features that are now just history. The first was 'Works Ambulances'. These were vehicles in company colours which provided transport from the works to the Accident Room for injured employees. The Tyneside heavy industries like the National Coal Board, Swan Hunters, Parsons and Armstrong all had ambulances. Was this service provided out of concern for staff welfare or did it reflect a dreadful health and safety record at the shop floor?

The second memorable feature was the frequency of sepsis, particularly hand sepsis, always Staphylococcal-based. Inevitably there were large collections of pus requiring surgical drainage. It was not uncommon to drain half-a-pint of pus from a breast or a leg. The classical features of lymphangitis were nearly always present. I suspect that the sepsis rate reflected the fact that there were essentially only three antibiotics available for general use, penicillin, tetracycline and sulphonamides, and that antibiotics were less commonly prescribed in primary care. And maybe the Staphylococcus has changed in nature, too?

Traditionally the house staff held a Christmas Concert which was held on a proper stage with a proscenium arch at the back of the infirmary canteen. At the last minute its organisation and directing was handed over to me, probably because at that point I was house officer for a female medical ward, which was a bit of a sinecure. Everyone else had busy jobs but in spite of that we managed to make a decent job of rehearsing. However, it was a requirement that a dress rehearsal was held in front of the House Governor, Professor Walder,and Matron, who acted as censors. I wasn't worried as I knew that there was nothing particular smutty in the script. They sat through the performance without comment, although since the script was a bit Monty Pythonesque I don't know how much of it they understood. This was probably not helped by the printed program which bore no relation to the actual content of the concert. Largely because in those days there were no PCs and laser/inkjet printers. So, our programme had to go to be typeset and printed a month before the concert date, and at that point we still didn't have a script. The censors did spot a rather blue joke which Jack Collin ad-libbed during one of his appearances. Only Professor Walder understood it, so the concert went ahead. We played to packed houses on both nights and raised nearly £100 for charity.

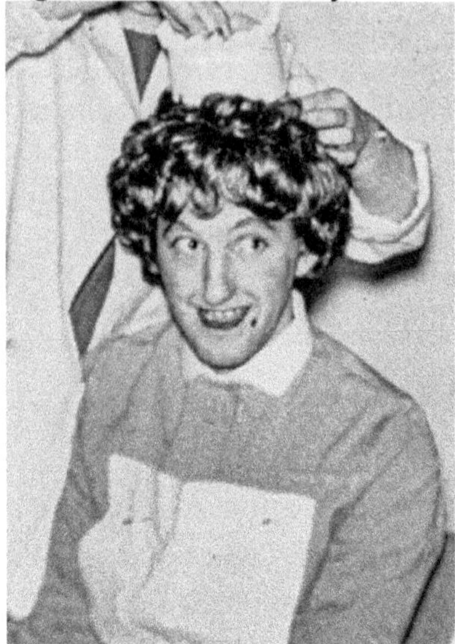

Tony Reed at RVI Xmas Concert 1968

At official social events at the RVI (Presentations, opening ceremonies, awards, etc.) a gin cocktail was always served. It was delicious and tasted innocuous so that it was very easy to slug down. Always with disastrous effects.

It was served at these events by the same ladies who waited-on in the junior doctors dining room and one day I persuaded Betty to get the recipe for me. She got matron's secretary to type it out.

GIN COCKTAIL

1 bottle of GIN

1 bottle of DRY MARTINI

2 tablespoons COINTREAU

1 bottle of LEMON SQUASH

The juice of four lemons.

Mix with about three ladles full of ice cubes. Make it in good time so ice cubes melt and there are small pieces of ice still floating around.

Below is a photo of Howard Young dressed in a staff nurse's uniform under the Christmas Tree in the Junior Docs Dining Room with Betty (left) and Doris (right).

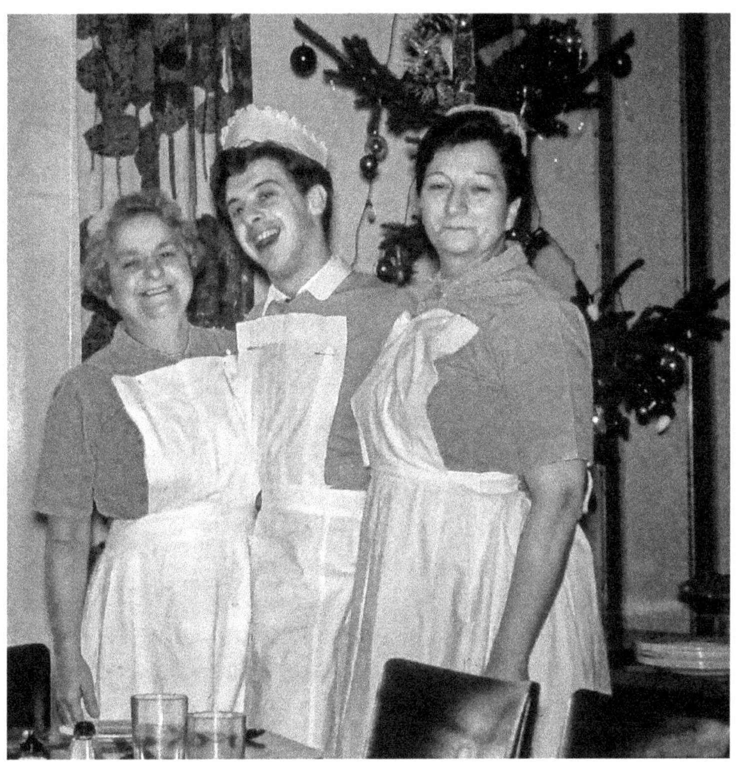

Old War Wounds

Junior surgeons at the start of their career were usually assigned to be the sole medical input to a variety of long-standing outpatient clinics. I found myself running the fortnightly bougie clinic at the RVI. I believe the bougie clinic was a hangover from Mr Feggetter's practice. He had honed his urology as a medic with the Desert Rats in North Africa in 1942 where, believe it or not, the invasion force landed at Bougie! The Newcastle clinic that I staffed was mainly attended by middle-aged men who had developed a urethral stricture as the result of venereal disease, often during the war. It was an open clinic, and they were allowed to turn up whenever they felt their stricture had narrowed down badly enough to cause them voiding difficulties.

These days I believe these strictures would be managed endoscopically under direct vision. Then it was a question of using a small calibre curved metal bougie (a Clutton's) to make an initial blind navigation through the stricture; then using progressively larger bougies to stretch the narrowed area. This had the potential for a lot to go wrong, particularly for an inexperienced junior. Not a lot for the man on the other end of the bougie, either.

All the men attending the clinic were old hands. They were in fear and dread of a new doctor turning up to run the clinic. New doctors usually had a steep learning curve, which potentially meant pain for the recipients. A good or bad reputation was rapidly gained, and it was not known for some of the men to walk out if a doctor with a bad name turned up.

The men all knew which size bougie they wanted you to start with, and the maximum size they could take. They knew the twists and turns of their stricture and some would direct you; "up a bit, doc", "to the left, now", "don't go there, doc", etc. Inevitably there was a little bleeding, but the real shame was for one of the attendees to turn up later that day at casualty with a clot retention. That news got round the infirmary rapidly. Fuel for a few jibes in the doctors' mess.

Talking out of your arse

In the mid-1980s I had just returned from a secondment at St Marks Hospital in London and was setting up a Colo-rectal service at the RVI. One of the aims was to develop an anorectal function lab to assist with the diagnosis and treatment of incontinence.

One crucial part of the work-up was to measure nerve conduction times. Those of you with long memories may remember that this involves sticking a concentric needle in the appropriate muscle and electrically stimulating the nerve which supplies it.

To assist me I had recruited Peter, a consultant neurophysiologist. The procedure involved inserting a fine needle into the anal sphincter and stimulating the pudendal nerve with a pad over the sacrum. These were the days before computers and the standard neuro-physiology kit was a cathode ray oscilloscope with a built-in speaker. This gave both a visible and an audible indication of the efficacy of conduction.

On this particular day we had successfully carried out two assessments and were setting up our third, a lady in her early fifties. We explained the procedure to her and put the sacral pad in place. Peter warned her he she was going to feel his needle and he gently placed it into the sphincter muscle and switched on the oscilloscope. Instead of hearing the usual hiss and crackle of muscle activity we heard some light music!

Peter looked embarrassed and made some adjustments to his equipment. The music continued. Were we overhearing it from next door? I did a quick recce and there was nothing audible in the corridor or adjacent room. I checked my bleep. No music there either.

Was it the equipment? Peter tried moving his apparatus and changing the layout of his leads in case they were acting as aerials. It made no difference. The band played on. Our patient was as intrigued as we were about the music and we had to explain that we would have to remove the needle and check the equipment before trying again. We did this and the lady was content that we have another attempt. The same again! By this time, we were all wondering if it was a radio broadcast, if so, which programme?

Peter re-positioned the needle to a different point in the sphincter without needing to re-puncture the skin. Again, the music rang out. But now our curiosity about the source of the music was satisfied. As the music came to an end, loud and clear from the speaker came the unmistakable tones of

"This is Jimmy Young and the JY prog. And here, hot of the press, is today's recipe and one of my favourites. Shepherd's Pie."

Needless to say, by this time all three of us were in stitches. Peter had several more attempts, but we had to apologise to the patient and abandon the procedure. Subsequently we were able to carry out the procedure on her without incident. Peter told me that he dined out on this story for months. I often wonder what the lady told her family.

Peter took his equipment back to the main lab and had it thoroughly tested but could find no fault with it. He told me that he thought some particular combination of circumstances had allowed the lady's anal sphincter to act as an aerial. Perhaps the orientation of the examination trolley or a combination of its materials or layout. Or the direction she was lying.

I didn't have the heart to ask if it would have been a ring antenna.

Alastair Scott Green

The week before Christmas

The phone rang as I was eating lunch. An agitated voice said, "Please come, doctor, Mr Smith has collapsed." The call was from the public phone box outside the village hall in a neighbouring village. As I drove to the village, I was recalling that Mr Smith had for three years together with the District Nurse devotedly cared for his bedridden wife following a major stroke until her death at home six months ago. A reception committee greeted my arrival, and I was ushered into the village hall kitchen where a body in a Santa Claus outfit was laid out on the floor. My certification of death was received in silence just as the noise of excited children's' voices permeated from the hall.

Newcastle Medical School training did not cover this emergency other than how to undress a body, but Santa Claus must never ever disappoint. There followed a magical hour as the locum Santa Claus listened to the Christmas wishes of twenty-three excited children. A Christmas to remember.

A Learning Curve

"You will be covering for Dr W for five days next week".

Dr W had for over thirty years been a single-handed GP in a village seven miles from our main surgery and my practice had for many years provided medical cover on the rare occasion when Dr W wanted time off. I say "my practice" but in fact I was three months into "an assistantship with view to partnership" so this was an opportunity to show my worth.

The waiting room doubled as the family dining room and eleven patients waited my arrival Having introduced myself, I took a note of their names and crossed the hall and entered the large Consulting room. The furniture comprised a roll top desk with a Windsor chair, two dining type chairs and an examination couch on which sat six wooden file drawers contains the Lloyd George patient notes. Having found the required notes, I deposited the drawers on the floor and commenced the surgery.

The majority of the presenting symptoms were for minor respiratory infections and my reluctance to prescribe antibiotics was not well received.

A further eight patients made an appearance, but several decided that they would prefer to await Dr Ws return rather than trust a youngster. After the last patient had left, I took the handwritten prescriptions into the adjoining dispensary in a converted garage and counted out the pills and filled the bottles ready for collection from the Housekeeper.
The Housekeeper had a list of six home visits in four different villages and she was able to give me directions and provide some background family history. Yorkshire folk are renowned for their friendliness and generosity and it was difficult not to cause offence by declining the offer of alcoholic refreshment at each location.
Returning for evening surgery I was surprised to find the file drawers back on the examination couch. After three days I asked the Housekeeper why she persisted in placing the drawers on the couch. "Dr W likes them there". I explained that I may need to examine a patient. "Dr W sends them home and goes to see them after the surgery".
That particular reason for a home visit was not covered by the Newcastle GP Vocational Training scheme but the likely provision of an alcoholic beverage might be persuasive.

A Journey

After retirement in 2004 I was the co-driver of a hired 30cwt Thames Carrier loaded with physiotherapy and special needs equipment on a 1500-mile journey from North Yorkshire via France, Belgium, Germany, Austria and Slovenia to Croatia.
Three months before I had been asked by a patient, a retired agricultural consultant, to assist him in procuring donations of equipment wanted by an Australian physiotherapist working voluntarily for the UK charity Hope and Homes for Children in Bjelave Orphanage in Sarajevo.
PHYSIONET was formed a year later and along with a network of enthusiastic volunteers collect, repair and pack donated medical equipment in the UK to help the less fortunate around the world. Amongst other organisations Rotary UK and Rotary International have supported and helped provide valuable trustworthy contacts abroad.

The base of the operation is a barn in North Yorkshire and there are collection hubs in the South East and South West. Collaboration with the Margaret Carey Foundation supplies wheelchairs to HM Prison service who repair and repaint as part of a rehabilitation programme.

We collaborate with other organisations including Form 4 Life, Jubilee Outreach Yorkshire Hope and Homes, Chernobyl Children and Breadline for part deliveries. Transportation is by 40 ft shipping containers and has been to destinations in 22 countries to date. In 2019, 8000 items with a value in excess of 1 million pounds were shipped to 14 countries. The 100th shipment was to Fiji in November 2020.

PHYSIONET, charity 1175932 was granted the Queens Award for Voluntary Service in 2018.

Mike Shadforth.

Check your facts!

I was recently qualified and working in a hospital serving a local mining community. I had been on call and it was busy, so that I didn't make bed until approaching 5am. I needed to be on the post take ward round at 9am and I planned to be up by 8.30 with time for a quick coffee before that. My best made plans were broken at 7.20 my phone ringing. It was my boss, who asked,

"How is Mr. Snookes?"

I had admitted Mr. Snookes the previous evening after he suffered a myocardial infarction and it now turns out that my boss knows him.

I said, "He is fine we will see him on the ward round",

and I got back to sleep for my remaining 70 minutes.

Arriving on the ward at 8.50 I decided to check on Mr. Snookes. His bed was empty! I returned to the ward office and asked the nurse there where he was.

"He died last night." said the nurse.

"Who certified him dead and why was I not called", I asked.

"I don't know", she responded, "I only came on at 8am".

I had no choice but to telephone my boss and admit that I had not been on top of my job and had thus misinformed him.

"Mr. Snookes is unfortunately dead", I said.

My boss was surprisingly understanding and said that he would call Mrs Snookes to commiserate.

I was only just off the phone call when sister appeared in the ward office. I took her to task, asking why her nurses had failed to call me when Mr. Snookes died. She gave me a perplexed look and said "Mr. Snookes isn't dead. His condition deteriorated and we transferred him to Coronary Care!"

I immediately called my boss again and fortunately got through before he had time to call Mrs Snookes. When I explained the situation again, I was asked if I perhaps thought it a good idea to go and see the patient! I agreed that sounded sensible and I set off down the corridor towards Coronary Care.

As I turned into the coronary care ward a crowd of individuals rushed past me and I realised they were the resuscitation team. They were heading of course to Mr. Snookes who unfortunately did not respond to the resuscitation.

Moral – be sure of your facts when communicating with the boss.

A case of Voodoo!

I was in my first medical job and I admitted an emergency case of anaemia. It was real anaemia with the haemoglobin, in old money, 3.9G per 100ml. For those who don't translate old money that is about 25% of what it should be and the patient, a man of 64, matched the colour of the bedsheets very well.

My medical training had been excellent, and I recognised the low white cell count and the large volume red blood cells indicating this was Pernicious Anaemia which would respond rapidly to an injection of Vitamin B12. I arranged this and explained to the patient who responded,

"I am going to die".

I assured him that he would be fine since we were doing the right things, but he persisted with the same line. Next morning, I repeated the blood count and as expected it had improved markedly. Despite that my patient insisted that he was going to die. I continued to feel otherwise.

After visiting that evening, I was asked if I would speak to my patient's son. The son was concerned that his father was convinced he was about to die. I explained the clinical facts and pointed out that his dad was wrong. His son was grateful for the explanation and we parted on good terms. The following morning at 10.15 my patient died. In communicating this to the family, I explained this was most unexpected and asked if we could be allowed to perform a post-mortem examination. The family agreed and at that examination no cause of death was found.

I recounted this event for several years as evidence that Voodoo does exist and if you are convinced you will die then indeed you will. Many years later I read an article in "The Lancet" warning clinicians to be careful when treating profound pernicious anaemia since the very rapid formation of new red cells mops up potassium and can lead to sudden death from hypokalaemia. That is not found at post-mortem since serum potassium rises on death.

Perhaps not Voodoo after all!!

Brian Sheridan

Medical Exams.

As a consequence of emigrating to Canada I inadvertently became experienced in the undergraduate dread, examinations. But perhaps it started with the interview for entry to Newcastle Medical School which I remember for only two things. 'What school do you go to?' Answer: 'Liverpool College', follow up question: "Where is that?" I became speechless, my only response was 'where the h… do you think it is?' Secondly, we found out later that the interview was never used in the selection process.

Some years later in the MRCP oral, the first question was, 'tell me about the dog as a vector of disease'. At least when I failed, I knew why, which was more than my brilliant Professor did when he revealed that he had failed the first time. Message learnt was that they were out to get you.

Next exam was the ECFMG, the necessary entry hurdle for the US. Held in an obscure and not very safe area in Liverpool. A trick I had heard rumored was that this was way of failing 'foreign' applicants who would be unable to find the location, used also in London at the Royal College, having an oral at Charing Cross and practical at the London Hospital a few hours later. My brilliance in finding the location was a good start but I had got the day wrong, a warning sign of a persistent life failure, repeated when booking my wife's return ticket from Brazil many years later. Six months later, on the correct day, I was as flummoxed by the oral English language component of this exam' as were the other 200 applicants, nearly all from 'abroad'. What was this strange drawling incoherent accent? Southern US.

Next up after a year in Canada was the LMCC. A National final year exam taken by all graduating students and foreign graduates (FMG's), needed for a licence to practice. This was held in the University hockey arena, thankfully after the ice surface had been removed. In excess of 200 supplicants held over two days, all multiple-choice questions. Unknown to we FMG's we were placed in the front rows and all U of Toronto students were behind us, positioned probably so as not to disturb the FMG's since they finished and left almost an hourly earlier. It was only a few years later when on faculty that I discovered there were courses with THE questions and answers being given out at some Canadian medical schools. Failure at this exam was unusual for Canadian graduates.

In case the great adventure to Canada did not continue I returned on vacation to take the RCPath exam in hematology, a mixed clinical and laboratory examination with a serious practical component. I arrived in Coventry to meet the other four examinees who were loaded down with their own microscopes, test tubes, pipettes and nervous excitement. I later learnt that my casual request to the examiners 'could I borrow a microscope?' was taken as a sign of superb self confidence. Little did they know of the bluffing of a native scouser. Not returning to Canada for a further few weeks I was eager to know the results, but they had been mailed to my home and the College could not give me the results over the phone. But they could tell me if I had a small or large envelope. Small was a pass, large had the application papers for a repeat.

On to the last one, the FRCP (Canadian) in hematological pathology. Having learnt from the Brits, this was also held in an out of the way place, Hamilton, Ontario. By then I had relocated to Nova Scotia and this required a 2-hour flight and 80 km bus ride. Unlike the RCPath (UK) exam the Canadian version had a significant practical component but no need to actually 'twiddle the tubes', clotting and crossmatching with dubious skill. The purpose seemed to be to find out how much you knew rather that what you did not know, a pleasant change. Colleges in Canada do not generate much income from exams and repeating has serious consequences to a relatively simple progression from trainee to staff/consultant employment.

One year later the Canadian Royal College needed a new examiner for my specialty! Who better? I was experienced, qualified and came from an area of the Country that was underrepresented. So back to Hamilton for a week in November in 1978. All Pathological Specialties were examined at the same time and the Chair of the full examining board was Dr Tom Muckle, now a Professor on the faculty of McMaster Medical School in Hamilton. He vaguely remembered me but could not remember why and I was not going to tell him that it was my habit of falling asleep in all his lectures and he had congratulated me at the time on my somnolence (see Paul Smith's recollection of lunches in the Haymarket Hotel).

Over the next 10 years I examined many of my future colleagues several of whom I failed at their first attempt, although our pass rates were close to 80%.

One, now a distinguished transfusion expert, actually thanked me for failing him as he knew his training had been inadequate and he did not feel confident to move on to a consultant position. Not all were as generous in their comments.

Nova Scotia is a beautiful, small Province which has an excess of Universities, a large military presence and a huge lobster industry. Not having many hematologists, I was volunteered to run the undergraduate course on 'Blood'. As well as the usual course components there was a need to set an examination – my specialty. At the time the University required short written answers as well as multiple choices. It was no surprise that handwriting skills were shortly to be abolished and spelling was 'how ever you feel dear, Canadian or English versions.' Answers did not always reflect what was taught and I was puzzled by the (male) student who stated that menstruation was 2x commoner in females, in a question on iron deficiency. Multiple choice questions replaced these short-written answers and in setting these MCQ's I relied on a lecture remembered from Newcastle pointing out tricks to pass with absolutely no knowledge of the facts. The right answer is never a), b) and d) are commonly correct etc. My questions had to be submitted to a review panel to see that they were not too esoteric. The panel rejected one of my questions since they thought I was being irreverent. The correct answer associated Thalassemia trait (one of the commonest genetic diseases in the World) with b) microcytosis and d) membership in a criminal organisation. They thought I was joking. But in my lecture, I had pointed out the connection of Italian Mafia organizations and thalassemia which is extremely common in parts of Italy. My last appointment in England had been as a research fellow in David Weatherall's Department, famous for their work on Thalassemia, and some of the Department's research funding had come from the March of Dimes Charity in New York, diverted to this important cause by some men with heavy accents and dark suites.

Paul Smith

Introduction to medical school

When you first walk into a room with a multitude of cadavers draped in white sheets your world changes forever. Well, what did you do today Paul? Well, I was dissecting this chap's head and when we had sawn off the top of the skull and his brains came into view ... well, it tends to stop conversations. Life can never be the same. Friends tend to look askance as you assume the mantle of a modern Burke and Hare.

The pervading aroma of formaldehyde seems to cling to your very person let alone your clothes so immune to the frequent hand washing so beloved of lady Macbeth. It takes months to realise you are not bathed in dissecting fluid, but your fingers are covered in Parker's Quink a wonderful ink leaking from your fountain pen and whose main constituent is formaldehyde. We were allocated our cadavers by our names. Ours was the S to T table. We were an eclectic mixture of resolute seriousness and indifferent irreverence. I recall five of us with great clarity the 6th I cannot place I fear we may have unwittingly dissected him.

Tom Barlow's wonderful drawings on the blackboard, George Abouna's two-and-a-half-minute attempt to say P…P… Parotid gland and sadly on reflection our complete inability to control our laughter. A matter of reflective shame And so my time in an anatomy lab came to an end or so I thought. Yes, later I applied for an anatomy demonstrator ship in Newcastle. I didn't get it. However, Reg Scothorne remembering I had helped with upper limb dissections in the Holidays told me to apply to Glasgow. I arrived to be interviewed by wee George Wyburn, the professor who simply said, 'Well laddie you're the boy Reg Scothorne has sent so when can you start?' Best interview ever!

Whilst there I started to go out with a girl I had previously gone out with four years earlier. Both of us had left the North East, she to join British united Airways flying here there and everywhere, including every now and then Glasgow! I was working hard for the primary FRCS so Anne would take a taxi to the University from her crew hotel and collect me from the anatomy Department.

This Department is huge and contains the Huntarian museum with all William Hunter's obstetric models and cast's and John Hunter's specimens. On leaving the Department we would walk past tins (large tins about 8ft by 4ft) labelled heads, thorax, lower limbs etc. Anne disbelievingly looked at the container labelled heads and was amazed to find it contained heads. You can tell I am a true romantic funnily enough we were married and remain so today!
Any attempts at romance never went smoothly as I was recently reminded by an ex-girlfriend at the wedding of a friend's daughter two years ago in Northumberland. This smouldering beauty (she still is) came over to reflect on our short liaison in 1966 terminated by my elective to the USA. She mentioned she would never forget the second date when I took her to an upmarket restaurant in an hotel just outside Durham, saying it was a rather sophisticated thing to do at our age and she would always remember it, particularly the hotel named Cock of the North. I rest my case Milud!

More Medical School memories
Pathology, biochemistry, pharmacology, and bacteriology passed in a blur eliciting no interest. Pathology lectures were at 2:00 PM given in a lecture Theatre that creaked like a ship at sea an impression compounded by the fact that lunch was a pie and a pint (? Singular) in the Haymarket. Lecture six was on syphilis I slept through--- it, the die was cast!
Then clinical attachments in the morning were followed by refresher systemic lectures in the afternoon and the clinical attachments were an introduction to real medicine and surgery in practise. The highlight was one month in the RVI with Henry Miller teaching us how to examine the nervous system, which he did with great skill. Both Henry Miller and Graham Teasdale looked to high heavens when they saw me recalling that I had been the first to pass out in the medical dinner the previous week.
Henry, the guest of honour, mentioned me in his after dinner-speech as displaying an aptitude for anaesthesia. It all started to go wrong when Brian Sheridan and I met at Dag Kremer's drinks party, he introduced us to Aquavit (more suited to running engines than to be ingested). Then it was off to the pub, followed by attendance at the free Sherry party organised by some misguided drug firm. I have never drunk Sherry since.

My abiding memory of the event (it is remarkable that any memory exists) was of throwing a potato at Tom Barlow just before losing consciousness.

Then being suspended between two obliging other students who dragged me to an area of lawn outside. My muscle tone was such that I flowed out of the wheelchair transporting me. Leaving at about 4:00 AM I was deposited outside Brian's flat, let in by Mba Onwukwe to find Sheridan prostrate on the sofa with a plastic bucket strategically placed close to his head again I was not alone.

When I awoke it had snowed and I was surrounded by about 20 white mounds from which pitiful groaning sounds emerged. I was not alone, only the first! I recall being taken to A&E for observation again a matter of regret and profound embarrassment, they have enough to do.

Henry had banked this memory. A delightful elderly lady from Two Ball Lonnen (only in Newcastle) came into his clinic suffering from Vertebrobasilar insufficiency. In a wonderful Geordie accent, she announced "Eee why doctor when I gans to look up I gan all dizzy like and I cawp awar." The latter meaning to fall over. Henry looked at our group saying, "Ladies and gentlemen I cannot vouch for you all, but I know at least one of you knows exactly how she feels". His gaze directed at me.

Years later doing neurology at Glasgow the first person I met on the wards was Graham Teasdale whose only comment was "Oh no not again".

St George's Morpeth

A long time ago in an era far, far, away the powers that be in the medical school, tiring of the rebellious students, dispersed them far and wide.

Some to the wilds of Northumberland others to the outer reaches of the empire with the worst destined for Sunderland, a wilderness inhabited by a tribe called the makers (Maccas!) The medical school retained the more sophisticated tribe of Packers, centrally. Some were sent below ground to work in pits mining coal, (a black substance whose only use is now confined to New Year's Eve), others to factories producing steel and glass and the most resistant sent to psychiatric institutions.

Thus, I found myself in Saint George's psychiatric hospital in Morpeth. Arriving there on my first morning I was assigned a seat in an ongoing group therapy session by an extremely helpful mental nurse, with instructions to come up with a diagnosis for the various participants. The three paranoid schizophrenics were easy to point out. He nodded sagely "Not bad, you picked well, managing to get all three of the consultant psychiatrists present, but still in my view you are pretty much spot on!"
Subsequent events suggested I could well have been correct. The director of the unit was experimenting with the use of LSD to enable repressed patients to relax and open up, he had clearly not heard of Lucy in the Sky with diamonds. A demonstration ensued.
The rebellious students were placed behind a sofa, an easel with painting materials organised and the female patient entered. She had already had her LSD and was now given intravenous sympathomimetic agents to enhance its effect. The reaction was immediate, as she amorously approached the retreating consultant until we watched her chase him round the room.
Each time he passed he shrugged saying "Normally she paints"! Eventually calm returned and she went back to her room. He, sitting disconsolately, admitted he never really wanted to be a psychiatrist but a professional football player, but he said their pay was so poor! I wonder what he would have chosen nowadays.
Thus, we all entered clinical medicine.

66

In the elective year 1966. Brian Sheridan and I decided on New York or as near as possible as we wanted to go to all the jazz clubs. The taxi drivers used to think we were crazy being dropped off in Harlem! We heard some fantastic jazz. The nearest we got to NY was St Luke's hospital in Bethlehem PA about 80 miles South West of the city. They actually paid us, remarkable, hence our choice. We had 99 day Greyhound unlimited tickets: cost $99! Every weekend we went to New York, to listen to jazz, slept in telephone kiosks in the Port Authority bus terminal, returning to Bethlehem in the morning.
At the end of our time there we took route 66 out to LA, then up to San Francisco and back to Bethlehem. Naturally going from one jazz club to another.

The elective had started with an Aer Lingus flight to Boston, where on our first day we were all invited to a barbecue held at the home of the president of the First National Bank of Boston. The next day Brian and I went up to Newport for the Jazz Festival prior to arriving in Bethlehem. Realising that UK 60s style haircuts, or the lack of them would not go down well we both had haircuts before going to the USA. On arriving in Bethlehem, we were collected by the CEO of the hospital (imagine that!) who drove us straight to the barbers where Bryan decided to go for broke and have the shortest of cuts. We met at the recent reunion and it has still not grown back.

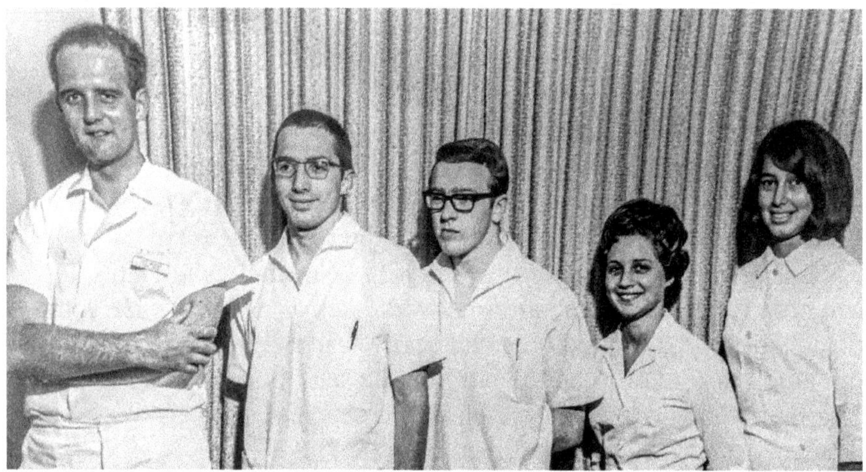

St Luke's hospital Bethlehem PA from left to right Horst Wengeler, Brian Sheridan, Paul Smith, Rose Marie Ripper +?

Back to Newcastle to finish our training with renewed enthusiasm for medicine, the American attitude was infectious. The next two years went quickly and suddenly it was 1968 and we were qualified. From then on you stood alone you had become responsible.
There are however certain things that you were never trained for and certification of death is one. Having been trained to keep people alive, certifying death is an odd position to be in. 'I'll just look for chest movements for a few more moments, maybe I'll cheque the heart again and look at the pupils again.' Then with a shaking hand you sign the certification of death, hoping when you leave the room the supposed corpse doesn't suddenly sit up and ask what the hell is going on?

Fortunately, this never happened to me, but something similar did. One of the registrars in Sunderland, a very bright guy but prone not to be overly helpful to the houseman became legless at one of the mess parties. He was taken down to the Mortuary and laid under a white sheet. When he awoke some hours later, he made his way through the hospital stark naked except for the white sheet and bumped into the night sister who apparently departed quickly.
He returned to his room which contained only a bare light bulb, all else had vanished. The window was open, and several floors below stood his bed…. vertically, he confided in me: (this was the only aspect of the experience that puzzled him) 'How come they threw it out of the window, and it landed end on with the bed clothes still in perfect condition?' He asked!
Clinical practice was different. Until now we had acquired lots of information but lacked experience, we were to learn that our preclinical work was simply the coat hanger on which to hang experience. Similarly, the layperson who acquires information on the Internet does not acquire knowledge, insight, or judgement, only if they are lucky facts. So, we knew about fibroids, but I remember the gynaecologist who fixed my gaze asking, 'Have you ever felt a fibroid boy?' 'No Sir.' 'Okay come with me' and after the appropriate examination 'Can you feel it?' 'Yes Sir' 'Good, now you will never forget what one feels like' and you never did.
Some of our clinical teachers had a real gift for embedding that experience into lasting knowledge. However, heart murmurs were way beyond me, maybe I had the head of my Littman stethoscope the wrong way round, but I could make no sense of them. I got the lub-dub of the normal beat but nil else.
Years later the same stethoscope was to cause much amusement. It was my surgical house job in Sunderland Royal Infirmary, where Malcolm Ayres and I alternated our house jobs. A patient had been admitted whom the surgical registrar and I suspected to possibly have a bowel obstruction with occasional loud and overactive bowel sounds. The consultant on call like to be informed of all admissions and was duly summoned. Being a man of immense presence and the singular ability to avoid speech unless absolutely necessary, he strode into the Ward to the bed, patient and awaiting medical staff. As he silently made to sit down on the absent chair, one was hastily found and suitably placed… prior to an impending disaster.

The right hand was thrust out, palm upwards awaiting the expected stethoscope.

Being closest I placed my Littman stethoscope in his hand, he looked at it for a good half minute (he had not seen one before) and proceeded to place it on the exposed abdomen. Head bowed, there he rested for a good two minutes before rising up declaring 'It's a silent abdomen'. Seeing the head of the stethoscope was not centred I realised no noise could be transmitted and taking it, adjusting it, I gave it back apologising that the head was not centred. At the second attempt bowel sounds made their presence felt. The maestro ascending from his purposeful posture announced bowel obstruction clearly! 10 years later I met the same registrar now a consultant in Louisville Ky when I was a hand fellow with Harold Kleinert -Small world.

I was privileged in Sunderland to work with Indian colleagues, most having suffered from discrimination but all taking such rebuffs on the chin, accepting it was the way of the world at that time. I found my colleagues, friendly, supportive, knowledgeable and learned so much from them. They taught you to accept responsibility, essential in medicine, especially if you are to be a surgeon. I was taught by them to be a thinking physician who could also operate. Not a bad philosophy. It avoids the stereotypic arrogant surgeon.

Give me a surgeon who questions, am I doing the right thing? Is there a simpler but just as effective method, and are we doing what is in the best interest of the patient? Ram Banerjee, Doctor Sinha and Mr Singh were my tutors.

As a houseman in six months, I undertook approximately 20 appendicectomies, six perforated duodenal ulcers and numerous minor other operations. I realised I wanted to do something involving my hands. Coming from Newcastle, neurology appealed so it had to be neurosurgery!

Neurology was wonderful anatomically based (remember Ramon Y Cajal mapping of neural pathways), intellectually stimulating, careful clinical examination revealing all. In those days' angiograms and air encephalograms were all that supplemented a clinical diagnosis. Then came the EMI scan -- put patient in tube -- get answer out, all the mystery vanished.

Glasgow in those days was the world centre for neurosurgery led by Professor Brian Jennett, whose textbook had received worldwide acclaim, Alistair Patterson, who had the largest series of cerebral aneurysms in the world and the unit was full of overseas registrars from the USA Canada etc.

However, neurosurgery was challenging. You could treat a disc, a meningioma (dicey), acoustic neuroma but aneurysm surgery could be perfect, but the patient could still succumb to vascular spasm four days later. Not much feedback for you as a surgeon.

During my time in the neurological unit in Glasgow we kept all head injuries who had been admitted unconscious under inpatient observation for one month, doing various tests such as caloric ear tests; the results of all this research became the Glasgow coma scale. The Ward was one of the early proponents of progressive nursing care. Immediately on entering the Ward you were in the ITU section with patients connected to inter cranial pressure monitoring and numerous other monitors, as you went around the U shaped Ward, the patients became more alert until the last area where they had recovered from severe head injury and surgery. It was in the latter area where things went pear shaped. One day Alistair Patterson (AP) was making rounds and as always was impeccably dressed in a pin striped suit with gleaming black shoes.

While discussing a recovering soldier who had a serious head injury, he became aware that the patient had presented his credentials and was quietly urinating on AP's shoes. The rest of us jumped back but AP remained immobile and unperturbed, calmly war watching the cascade of urine hitting those gleaming shoes. Once the flow ceased AP turned to the Ward sister saying

‘Mr. Johnson appears a touch frontal lobeish today sister’ and moved on to the next bed.

He was equally calm in surgery, one of the finest technical surgeons I have ever seen. Neurosurgery did not have the interest that neurology held-- at the end of my time there I was experienced in three things-- opening skulls, removing infected bone flaps and revising VP shunts. My future was elsewhere.

My next rotation was with Athol Parkes, a renowned hand surgeon, meticulous in documenting his examinations, careful history, clinical diagnosis, anatomically based surgery, and it really mattered who did the surgery. My future was set!

He could test every muscle in the upper limb in two minutes. The film of this is still held by the British society for surgery of the hand. Athol was a petrolhead, two wheels or 4. He used to bike down to BSSH council meetings in London from Glasgow. He had two speeds, parked or flat out. Probably the only council member to walk in wearing bike leathers and with a face like a panda.

On one occasion the engine of his BSA seized, being Athol, he rang the MD of the company who sent a van to collect him and bike, the bike had a new engine put in while Athol was treated to lunch. On another occasion having arrived at the elective orthopaedic hospital in Killearn about 20 miles outside Glasgow, Athol proudly announced to the Prof that he had shaved 45 seconds of his best time. The Prof's response, 'Tell me Athol what do you plan to do with your extra 45 seconds?'

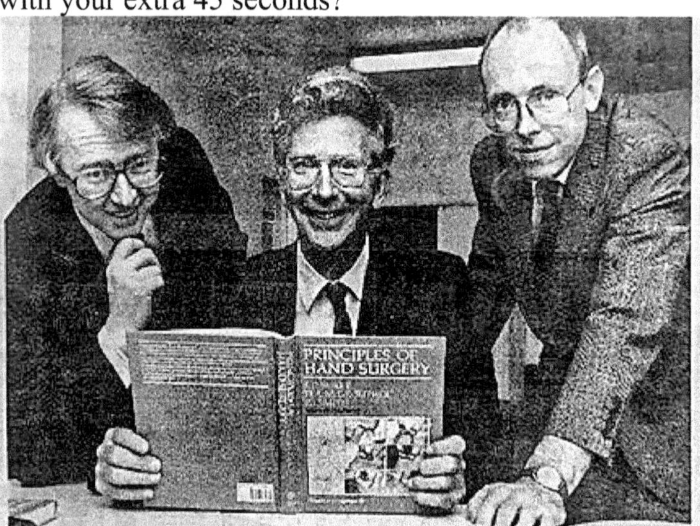

Left to right: Paul Smith, Frank Burke, and Prof. Angus McGrouther

Wear-link surgeons return

THREE of the country's top surgeons, who learned their skills in Sunderland, returned to the district for the launch of their first book.

Professor Angus McGrouther, plastic surgeon at University College Hospital, London, Paul Smith, consultant hand surgeon at Great Ormond Street Hospital, London, and Frank Burke, consultant hand surgeon at Derby Royal Infirmary chose Sunderland to launch their book "The Principles of Hand Surgery".

Both Mr Burke and Mr Smith are the sons of doctors and were born in Sunderland and did their hand surgery training in the area.

Prof McGrouther came to Sunderland as a plastic surgeon and helped develop the district's reputation for hand and plastic surgery.

Ram Banerjee, accident and emergency consultant at Sunderland District General Hospital, organised the book launch and a seminar on hand surgery at the hospital, said: "These three men are eminent in their profession and have achieved national fame."

Barbara Spencer

Medical Reminiscences

As a student I was working on a surgical ward. A man presented with a most embarrassing problem. His wife was nearing the end of her pregnancy. Marital relationships were off limits and so he was looking for other means of gratification. He came up with the idea of using a clothesline and inserting it into his bladder. The only problem was that the line became tangled in his bladder and he was unable to retrieve it. There were yards of it! The surgical registrar was dumbfounded and gave him some alternative advice post-operatively!

When working in my first practice a man presented with tonsillitis one morning. I gave him the usual advice along with a prescription for antibiotics. I was on call for the afternoon and was somewhat surprised to receive a desperate call from him because he was no better. He had had the first dose of medication about 3 hours previously and wanted a home visit (those were the days!). I said that I would call in on my way to evening surgery. When I arrived at his house, I was greeted by an apologetic but thankful patient. He had improved considerably. As a consequence, he gave me a bunch of magnificent chrysanthemums that he had grown. He was clearly an expert in growing the flowers and took great pains with the inflorescence. They were a sight to behold in his garden.

There was a renowned psychiatrist called Dr Fank Lake in Nottingham. He had become involved with St John's College, where Anglican priests trained. He realised that the "modern" trend for priests' wives to be more independent and less involved with parish work was causing strains on the clergy. The parishioners did not accept the changes that were taking place nor that priests might have difficulty with coping.

As a result, he set up courses in Clinical Theology, which became a national organisation, and which he opened up to members of the public as well as the priesthood. He then went on to form a group of people which he trained in counselling, long before it became recognised as such.

Through a friend I was asked to join the group and did so very uncertainly. The sessions were informal and, eventually, we were each asked to take on clients. The consultations were to take place at a centre in the city.

An appointment had been arranged for a lady to see me, but the day was a Bank Holiday. She insisted on seeing me, saying that she was desperate and would see me at my house. Under great pressure I agreed. When she arrived, she had flowing long hair, dark purple, swirling clothes and was incredibly thin. She reminded me of pictures of witches. My dog went to greet her but rapidly turned round with her tail between her legs, which added to my impression! The story she told me was lengthy and very strange. I began to wonder how much was factual. I offered her a cup of tea at the end. My dog came into the room but went all of the way round the outside and then out again as fast as she could instead of approaching the lady in her usual fashion. My husband thought the lady was odd too. I found it interesting that a normally friendly and very sociable dog should be so wary of a person she had never met before. However, the skills I learnt from Frank Lake proved to be invaluable in General Practice. He was an enthusiastic, empathetic doctor and excellent teacher who was keen to explore new ideas. He was not at all like the stereotypical psychiatrist.

Many years later I asked a student to interview the next patient on his own. When I joined them, I realised why it had taken so long. The patient was a man in his 30's and presented with anxiety symptoms, amongst others, and was keen to tell his story. I suggested that we should refer him on, but he was insistent that he did not want that because he had seen "everyone".

I agreed to continue to see him, and it became apparent that he had a dreadful obsessive compulsive disorder. Over time he recounted his difficulties of getting up in a morning, parking his car, and so on. Everything had to be done in a particular sequence and perfectly, otherwise he would have to start again. Sometimes he struggled to get to his appointments on time.

One day he rang from the village phone box to say that he might be late. I told the receptionist to tell him that I would not wait beyond a certain time, as I thought it would be good for him. I was astounded when he arrived almost to time but out of breath and bright red in the face.

He had run all the way from his village – 5 miles away – because his car would not start. I felt a bit guilty! He did improve over time. We injected some humour into his exploits and that helped. Eventually he moved out of the area, but his new GP told me that he was still managing reasonably well.

I liked all aspects of Practice and, being in a semirural area, enjoyed using various surgical techniques. A GP from a local practice had decided to change medical careers but, in the process, did some locum work. He came to help out and walked into the treatment room as I was incising an ingrowing toenail. He looked over my shoulder and muttered.

“Chinese torture!”

A man rang the receptionist many years ago and said he thought he’d been given the wrong prescription. It was for Lobak, but his problem was his upper back and shoulder!

One night I was called to a house in St Anne’s, Nottingham. It was not my practice area, so I did not know it very well. My husband was aware of the area’s reputation and insisted on driving me there! The front door was at the top of a flight of steps and recessed. When the door was opened the passageway was lit by the dimmest light possible. The outline of the figure at the door proved to be a small man who signalled me to follow him to the end of the passage and into a bedroom. Then he left. It all felt a bit eerie. The light in the bedroom was marginally better than that in the hall. Apart from the bed there was just a wardrobe with some things on top and no carpet on the floor, which was tiled. The bed was covered with a higgledy-piggledy pile of different coloured dirty looking blankets and at one end there was a lady. She recounted her story. Then, as I was about to examine her, different parts of the blankets moved and out came several cats. I was not expecting that! It was clear she had a closer relationship with the cats than with the man. I had to go downstairs to speak to him and was struck by how difficult their circumstances were. The obvious poverty and lack of understanding were making a significant contribution to the way they managed their lives, and they seemed to think that was how it should be. The cats provided the affection they needed.

One winter we had early snow which stayed for a few weeks. A patient rang to ask for a visit. The weather was too bad for them to come to the surgery. It was suggested that the conditions would be exactly the same for one of the doctors! Still a visit was required.

In my first hospital job I was on call at Christmas. I was surprised to find that I was expected to join several members of staff and visit most of the wards – for a sherry at each one!

My main wards were surgical, and the men's ward had a delightful but earnest Charge Nurse.

Some of the doctors and nurses got together and decided to play a trick on him. In Casualty, someone was bandaged up from top to toe and limbs plastered. A drip was erected. I was told to tell the Charge Nurse that a man was being admitted and that he had horrific injuries. The Charge Nurse started rushing around getting a bed ready on the ward. The "patient" was wheeled in. It was a little while before the penny dropped. He took it in good part, fortunately, and the other patients on the ward thought it was hilarious. A good tonic. Then we all had our Christmas lunch on the ward, using makeshift tables. How times have changed!

One of my partners was a bit like Siegfried in "All Creatures Great and Small". He had lots of energy and enthusiasm. If his surgery was running late or he felt stressed he would sometimes commandeer another consulting room so that the next patient would be ready when he was. One day, in his usual hurry to be away he had asked an elderly lady whom he knew well to wait in the other room. 2 hours later, when he had left the surgery long since and along with most of the staff, she emerged and asked the receptionist if she thought the doctor had forgotten her! The stoicism of some of the rural population is remarkable at times and her generation had great respect for their doctor.

My partner, Bob Berrington, was Regional Advisor for General Practice. He was quite a character, full of enthusiasm for new ideas and progress in General Practice.

As you may imagine, our practice was at the forefront of many of the changes. It was semirural but over the past years there have been huge developments of housing especially for one of the commuter villages.

Bob had a great rapport with his patients and had a fund of stories. We had many debates in the 80's about how General Practice should develop. We were earnest about accountability, assessment, and best practice.

However, I remember one of the debates and arguing that what was being assessed was what was measurable i.e., quantity rather than quality. I still do not know how to assess the latter. Patient satisfaction was discounted because they would be biased. Time management became important, understandably, but patients and their problems do not fit in boxes.

An example of an outcome that was difficult to measure is as follows. A tall and well-built man came to see me. I had never seen him before. To say he was on edge was an understatement. He paced the waiting room hitting the palm of one hand with the fist of the other and continued to do the same when he came into the consulting room. He was feeling angry about something too.
I suddenly felt a bit vulnerable when I realised that he was between me and the door. I managed to discover his problem and continued to talk to him. Gradually he calmed down and was able to sit down. At the end of the consultation, I asked him if he would like a prescription and he said "No", he'd be alright now. I had given him some understanding and strategies, together with some time, and that was all he needed. He did not even need a follow up! Bob spent time with patients when they needed it too, and they appreciated it.
Once I was inveigled into being the MO for Brands Hatch Racing Circuit when the orthopaedic registrar who usually did it became unavailable. Over the phone he was quite reassuring. BMW saloon cars were being demonstrated and he was sure I would have nothing medical to do and if there was a problem there would be help at hand! Potential customers would be driving.
In the observation tower I watched some extremely fast driving and as a thank you I was driven round the circuit in the car of the mechanic who had been my minder throughout the day.
I had only been qualified about four months! To say I was apprehensive would be an understatement but the guys looking after me were very kind and encouraging…...but all they gave me to settle my nerves was a cup of tea. The car I was in was fast but nowhere near the power of the ones that had been driven earlier by the clients and reps. Seeing my anxiety he took me round at a steady 70-80 mph, which was fast enough for me, but nowhere near some of the speeds of earlier in the day.

My first practice had no appointment system and we visited virtually everyone who requested a visit. On 3 days a week we had no afternoon surgeries, just morning and evening. I lived outside of the practice area so I would often shop in the village in the afternoon, at different times depending on how many visits I had.

The butchers, the younger owner and his assistant Cyril who was in his in his fifties, had a great sense of humour and were intrigued by what I did as a job. I wouldn't tell them, so they tried to guess. Each time I went in they had another suggestion, each time I said "No". Eventually they decided that I must be a bricklayer. It should be remembered that women doctors were very much in a minority.
When I had my first child I decided to resign from the practice and subsequently was asked to do locums in my village practice. It was very different - 5 minute appointments and patients were called via the intercom.
One day, after a couple of years or so, I called the next patient and Cyril presented in the doorway. The look on his face was a picture. It took him a little while to recover, and I had a struggle to stop myself from laughing. He was quite relieved that his "problem" was above the waist! Going into the butchers after that was even more delightful.
I served on several boards and committees and gained an insight into how things do and don't work in the NHS at different levels. When I was appointed to the Cambridgeshire Health Commission the first meeting was in November.
The discussion became relatively heated at one point about waiting times. It was clear that one or two there had vested interests. They were adamant that the waiting times for admission to hospital had to be reduced and just could not understand why it was so difficult. It was simple maths! Eventually, I said that, whilst it was a laudable idea, there were times when other priorities should win out.
I gave the example that during the coming 2-3 months there would be people requiring beds because of chest infections, winter accidents and so on. I thought they should be the ones admitted to hospital if necessary and that it wouldn't matter so much if people with less urgent conditions waited a bit longer and cited varicose veins!
I also explained how stressful it could be to all concerned to find beds, especially in the winter months. They were rather surprised because they hadn't realised how difficult it can be at times to juggle the response to the demand for beds. The Coronavirus has highlighted this once more.

On the same committee there were a number of academics from Cambridge University. One was an astrophysicist, and we were on a sub-committee. She was cross and bemused by the fact that not all GPs practised in the same way nor offered the same facilities.
I had said that we offered a certain service in our surgery and she wanted to know why she could not access it in hers. She had no appreciation that we all had different experiences during our medical training and, as with all people, different skills and strengths.
We were also the Board that was involved in the Child B case. I had been a fan of Panorama until then. Part of our Board meeting was filmed but the edited version did not show the balance of the debate!
When the Commission was disbanded a new Board was formed and a Social Worker appointed as CEO. He caused relative havoc and then went to the West Country. He recognised that he was not well-liked by GP's, so I hope he learnt from his experience with us. I wondered if he came to your area.

More Medical Memories

One night, when I was not on call, there came an urgent knock on the front door accompanied by ringing of the doorbell. It was about 2 am. My husband went to see who was there and called me to go down too.
I was more than surprised to find my Nurse Practitioner accompanied by a police officer. It seems that she had been asked if she knew a doctor nearby and thought of me. She hadn't got my phone number to hand so they took a shortcut and walked to my house. They wanted me to go and see someone who was badly injured on a nearby road. My husband decided to drive us – a longer route but more comfortable as there was a deep frost on the ground and did not take more time. When I arrived at the scene, I found a man lying in a pool of blood by the roadside. On examining him I found that he was not only lifeless, but his throat had been cut from ear to ear. I wasn't sure why I had been called, given that the ambulance was already there, but apparently they needed permission from me to move him!
It transpired that the man was in the USAF and had been to a party nearby. He had paid a bit too much attention to the wife of another USAF serviceman and as they were going home the aggrieved husband had slit the man's throat and thrown him out of the car onto the grass verge.

My Nurse Practitioner had been baby-sitting in another village and had noticed him on her way home. She decided that it was not safe to stop and rang the police when she arrived home. They asked her to return to the scene and meet them there.

She had a dreadful time of it. Not only was she a key witness and had to give detailed statements but she had to attend the trial, which took place at a USAF base over 80 miles away and took several days. It was a most unpleasant and stressful experience for her. The time involved was enormous. Thankfully all I had to do was give a detailed statement. I often walk past the place where the body was found and find that the memory comes back unbidden.

When I joined my second practice, I found that one of the nurse practitioners (they weren't called that then but did far more than the usual practice nurse) was running a weight clinic. I was asked to become involved and spoke to the group – all ladies who had been trying to lose weight for varying lengths of time. I gave them advice and targets and initially they did well.

Then, as was the norm, their weight plateaued. I was put under pressure to *do* something! A week or two later a flyer came to the surgery.

It was advertising a course in hypnotherapy at Cambridge University and was being run by doctors. I remembered that the GP with whom I had spent a couple of weeks as a student had used the technique for pregnant ladies. He had promised to demonstrate it, but we ran out of time. With that in mind I went to the course, feeling very sceptical and uncertain. However, I was impressed by what I learnt. When I returned to work, I was asked repeatedly when I was going to try it out, but I didn't feel confident! It was the time when complementary medicine came to the fore. A patient came to see my partner and asked him if he knew anyone who used the technique – and, of course, he said yes! The patient was a scientist and reputedly they make the most difficult subjects, but I couldn't refuse. With trepidation I spoke to him and taught him how to use it for himself. When he came back, he was full of enthusiasm at its effectiveness. So, now, I had no excuse but to use it for the weight clinic.

They all came one Friday morning, some were sceptical, others had open minds. I explained that I couldn't *make* them lose weight, nor do anything which was against their will/nature.

Part of the programme was to introduce suggestions about exercise and healthy eating. They came back each week and after the sessions would have some conversation. One lady was a Home Help. She cycled from one client to the next in the village. One day she was stopped by someone who asked why she always *pushed* her bike these days and no longer cycled. She was diabetic and enjoyed a French coffee every Friday evening. She recounted that she no longer enjoyed the coffee, and in fact, it made her feel nauseous! She did not make the connection and was still a bit dubious about the effectiveness of the sessions, although most of the others did! For quite a while the group continued with some success.
I still felt hesitant about admitting that I used hypnotherapy but went on other courses and became more confident. Consequently, there were some interesting success stories, especially for anxiety and phobias, which could not be the result of just giving people more time, although that was important too. What a pity quality time spent with patients isn't valued in the same way as quantifiable measures which meet various targets. It could save the NHS a great deal of money.

Peter Tate

Dad, Henry Miller, and John Walton.

My first limited experience with illness and faulty communication came via my father. He was a single-handed GP in South Shields working from a damp basement surgery in Beach Road. He became slower, felt indefinably below par and on occasions, embarrassingly, slurred his words. This was1960, he was 43, a heavy smoker (always the red, flat-packed Du Maurier) and no mean gin drinker with a history of a severe depressive episode requiring inpatient admission and ECT a decade earlier. There is a cartoon of him at this time, drawn by the artist of the Shields Gazette.

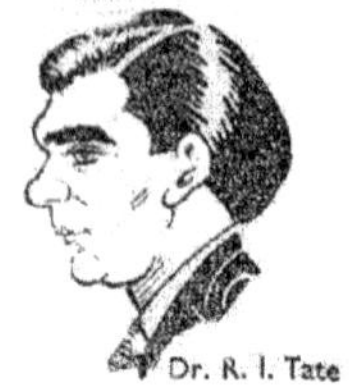
Dr. R. I. Tate

His very good friend was Henry Miller, then Dean of Newcastle Medical School, and one of the most admired Neurologists in the country. They had been at Durham together and kept in touch. Henry was a bon viveur, a larger-than-life theatrical character, with immense charm and wit. Dad consulted him about his symptoms. Henry was not impressed and rang my mother without father's knowledge, to say that dear Ivan was getting more hypochondriacal as the years went on and should cut down on the gin and fags. Mother was unimpressed but Dad had a stab at cutting down and soldiered on. Nearly three years went by and, by some fluke or misjudgment on Newcastle University's part, I started there on 2nd September 1963, my seventeenth birthday.

I had been away at boarding school, but once back at home it was obvious that Dad was increasingly unwell but pig-headedly soldiering on; his friend had told him he was ok so he would get through it.

We persuaded him to go back, Henry was unsure and sent him for a second opinion from his deputy and rapidly rising star John Walton.

After a couple of tests and a brief admission the diagnosis of Myasthenia Gravis was made. I think Henry was mortified. I do know that in my entire time at University he never spoke to me once, claiming later that he did not know I was Ivan's son. He did you know.
I met the by then Sir John Walton 30 years later when he became warden of Green College in Oxford and his daughter became our practice nurse in Abingdon.

The Club A'Gogo.

The club A'Gogo was very near the Medical School in Percy Street (properly pronounced Porsey). It was on the second floor of the Handyside Arcade in the Haymarket, now demolished. It was founded by that extremely dubious character Mike Jeffery and in early1964 the resident band was The Allan Price Combo of course soon renamed The Animals. The club flourished during our time at Uni and went out of business as we left. Newcastle students were treated as members on production of our Union Card.
Frankly, it was a bit rough, exciting, full of smoke, awful hamburgers and smelt of stale beer and Brut. Still looking too young to be in the sixth form, I finally managed to persuade a girl to go out with me and decided to take her to the club. She lived in South Shields and I picked her up in my Babe Magnet, my mother's Ford Popular.
She looked stunning, Judith Mc something, and was wearing a tight black sweater and extremely short skirt. All my Christmases had come at once. Even better (which she must have known) was the club's lighting system, which was ultraviolet light which made the girls underclothes fluoresce.
The night was a special night, there was a lot of such nights in that magical dump. Bo Diddly was over from the US of A on Eric Burden's invitation and it was a blast. They tried out their soon to be famous 'House of the Rising Sun' and other great blues numbers. Judith and I were sweatily dancing with gay abandon and I thought I was James Bond.
During a lull, a chap tapped me on the shoulder and asked if the pair of us would like to go backstage to meet the performers. Seemed a great idea…it wasn't.

Of course, Eric Burden had spotted Judith, who was a stunner, and way out of my league. It soon became apparent that three was a crowd. I waited some time, but she never did reappear, eventually I was told my services were not required to get her home, and never saw her again from that day to this.

A lucky policeman.

In 1966 a young bright Durham graduate became a consultant endocrinologist at the RVI, his name was Reg Hall. He went on to become an eminent and important professor and died too young, but my story relates to him being an acutely observant and exceptional clinician. One day he was driving his little Austin down Northumberland St to the extremely busy and complex junction at the bottom. In those days this busy junction was patrolled by a regular traffic policeman on a raised dais. Reg had noticed this man on several occasions and wondered about him, on this day he made up his mind and stopped right next to the policeman, who naturally was disconcerted and initially angry. He thrust a card into the white gloved hand, saying 'I am Doctor Reg Hall from the RVI, I think you have a condition that I could help you with and I would like you to come to my clinic at the hospital tomorrow.' Fortunately, the policeman did exactly as requested as his prominent jaw and muscular figure that had been admired by many had been recognised by Reg as a classical example of acromegaly, an over secretion of growth hormone. This was confirmed by various tests and the policeman's life was prolonged and improved by a successful operation on his pituitary adenoma.

The Pharaoh, South Shields General, December 1968

By the 1960's the British Raj was a rapidly fading communal memory, a thing of thick ruby port voices on late night radio programmes discussing tiger shoots. The sub-continent was divided into the two Pakistans, East and West, Muslim in creed, with India in the middle now populated mainly by the Hindu and the Sikh. Independence had been granted as recently as 1947 but the only legacies remaining to the average Englishman were dark curry houses with furry wallpaper and golden elephants on the walls, and the National Health Service.

At this juncture in history all general hospitals in ordinary unglamorous towns were staffed almost exclusively by Doctors from the sub-continent. The plum consultant jobs were still mostly in the hands of UK graduates, but the Senior Registrar, Registrar, Senior House Officer and Houseman posts were 95% Asian. The British graduates clustered into the Teaching hospitals, the centres of excellence, bastions of privilege and prejudice where dark faces were rarely seen and then only at monthly district meetings.

The South Shields General Hospital was an old workhouse; it was not in any way glamorous and had only one white houseman, me. My father Ivan was a General Practitioner in the town, and it was his longstanding friendship with a local general surgeon and director of Newcastle United, Bobby Rutherford, that had led me back to the old hospital to be apprenticed to him for six months.

It was the time of the war between India and Pakistan over disputed areas of Kashmir, the mix of doctors then working in the hospital was approximately two thirds Pakistani and one third Indian. Relationships were fraught and tension was high. This was not helped by the communal living arrangements of the doctors; we were all obliged to live in a self-contained stockade like edifice situated a hundred yards from the main hospital and known to all as 'The Ranch'.

As the tension built up the rival groups tried to cope by enlisting humour, but religious and patriotic rivalry is no laughing matter and quickly the two groups polarised absolutely into separate dissenting factions mutually loathing the other.

The demarcation of living room space and use of dinner tables became rigid with unspoken but unbreakable rules clearly understood by all.

The various medical and surgical teams began to suffer especially those with a religious mix, intermediaries such as myself passed messages and many jobs went undone. To make matters worse each faction followed the daily news of the war in the newspapers and from the BBC news bulletins with a fanatical intensity, celebrating successes without restraint, each time increasing the gap between them and raising the level and intensity of the recriminations.

During this period there were only three non-combatants living in the Ranch.

I, a wet behind the ears agnostic Geordie; Freddie a Patan from Afghanistan whose father was a chief and he was heir apparent; and Khurshid Qasimayya, a young big Egyptian doctor, with a physique like a Nubian wrestler and a similar command of the English language. In the early stages of the conflict, it was Freddie who helped most. He had no truck with either India or Pakistan. His revered forebears had a long and proud record of fighting all comers from Alexander the Great to the British, (and of course more recently the Russians, the Americans and the British again), and it was his solemn boast that though his fierce tribesmen had occasionally lost a skirmish they had never truly lost a war.
Freddie was a wiry, dark aquiline man with thick black grizzled hair, and quick searching eyes that demonstrated to those who wished to see them glimpses of his cat like intelligence and warrior's rumbustious sense of humour, unusual on the sub-continent. In keeping with his persona, he was possessed of an acute awareness of the feelings of others, detecting subtle nuances where others would just see hatred.
If Freddie followed a God, he never told the rest of us, but he did attempt to stop the others being consumed by their own Gods. He seemed to decide that if he could not stop the real war, he could at least help make the war being waged in this little part of Tyneside look as ridiculous to the combatants as it did to those uninvolved. He set about regaling each side systematically with blood chilling tales of his peoples' sufferings, their massacres, their triumphs and their many Pyrrhic victories. He adjusted the tales only a little depending on his audience.
To the Indians he described the deeds of his warriors against the Sikh and the Hindu and to the Pakistani it was against the Muslim of the plain.
Always of course the Patans were superior in every department, one musketted knife wielding terror from the mountains bettering at least ten Indians or Pakistanis in every bloody encounter, always outgeneralling and outlasting their puny opponents.
Initially irritation was the dominant emotion in the opposing camps when Freddie tried his simple strategy but gradually his humour, his persistence and his underlying sense of the ridiculous, backed by centuries of futile suffering, began to tell on the entrenched belligerence of the two sides.

The atmosphere became less charged, even an occasional smile could be seen and jokes in football metaphors began to appear along the lines of 'India 2 Pakistan 1 but it's gone to extra time'. The mess was still not a pleasant place to live in, but Freddie had made it bearable.

Khurshid, the Egyptian, was an altogether different kettle of fish. He was one of those human beings forever doomed to be in the wrong place at the wrong time doing the wrong thing for the wrong reasons. In a brief acquaintance this can be almost endearing but living with such a ninny, especially one with no command of the language of the land could become somewhat trying.

He was not helped by choosing as his little part of England to stay in and gain experience South Tyneside; an area with distinct customs and an impenetrable dialect which could only be understood by true natives born and bred Geordies.

The aforesaid Geordies are by and large a good natured wry humoured group who could not cope easily with a name like Khurshid Qasimayya, in no time of his arrival at the hospital he was christened 'The Pharaoh' (Fair-O in the dialect).

Within a few days of his starting to work as a front of house casualty officer he was confronted by a distraught young father pulling him into a cubicle with the desperate message of:

"Docta, Docta kum quick like. Wor bairn's fair felled an he's gorra load of blebs under his oxters an' he's burnin' up. Wor hen's beside hersel' with frit."

One week at the South Tyne Polytechnic night school on colloquial English was insufficient for him to have even the faintest clue of what the father was talking about; a large world weary casualty sister of the type they sadly don't seem to make any more translated slowly for him.

"What Mr Jones is trying to tell you Doctor is that he is worried about his little boy who has a rash of spots under his armpits and who seems to have a high temperature, his wife is very worried too. I think he has a mild dose of the Chickenpox." He only lasted six months as you will see but his English never did improve, forever held back by the vernacular. He must have returned to his ancient homeland with confused tales of this strange tribe of people living on the banks of a famous river whose customs and language were indecipherable to civilised nations. Perhaps he had unwittingly discovered how the Emperor Hadrian probably felt.

The Geordie people held a deeply schizophrenic view of the foreign doctors entrusted to look after them. They saw themselves as a separate tribe that just happened to live in North East England, so to some extent the Indians, Pakistanis even the Pharaoh were acknowledged as members of just another tribe like Scotsmen or Scousers or even Brummies. It was the older people whose deeply entrenched small town racism proved a bigger barrier to communication with the foreign doctors than any language barrier. My great aunt Vera was one of these.

At the time of this story, she was 80 years old, a small, wizened spinster who had been a lady's hatter in the town for 50 years, a business she had run with her eccentric sister Nellie. Neither had married, both had future husbands killed on the Somme and had accepted that men were not for them. It was rare that any man ventured into their little powdered shop and those who did were soon shooed away. Vera, the last and tiniest of a litter of 15, was known colloquially as 'the poke shakings' and had her left kidney removed on the kitchen table in extremely primitive and unhygienic circumstances at the age of 5. The doctor had solemnly given her but a few weeks to live; Vera did not however have another day's illness till her 80th year, demonstrating clearly the medical profession's fallibility when predicting the future.

Pain in the lower part of her belly and a fear of dying had brought great aunt Vera into South Shields General. She had lasted for a week at home, but the onset of vomiting and a complete blockage of the bowel finally ended her resistance and now she lay clutching the sheet to her chin peering fiercely at the group of doctors at the foot of her bed.

The tale was related to me later by Freddie the Patan, the Senior Surgical Registrar.

The Pharaoh was cowering at the back of the group as far away from the old lady as he could go while still maintaining contact with the ward round.

"Stay away, the lot of you." squawked an obviously cornered Vera, "It's not yer faces I object to it's yer black hands, and HIM" a white stick like arm shot out from under the sheet and pointed unequivocally at the cowering Pharaoh, "He's a menace, a loony. He's not a Doctor he's a monkey, all he talks is gibberish and he tried to stick a needle into my belly, well I'm not having it and that's final."

She pulled the sheet tighter to her chin and glowered at the assembled group daring them to make a move. Freddie took a pace forward; Vera shrank away up on her pillow.

“Gerroff.” It was a standoff.

Freddie turned to the ward sister for an explanation of the old lady’s aggression towards Dr Qasimayya, not wishing to risk a long incoherent conversation with the man himself. Sister cast her eyes heavenwards.

“I am afraid neither Miss Scarfe nor Dr Qasimayya understood much of what said. Miss Scarfe objected to him trying to examine her and screamed out loud when he put his hand on her tummy. I believe this somewhat unnerved Dr Qasimayya, for when he tried to take some blood from Miss Scarf’s arm, he tripped yelled and stabbed the syringe into her just below the umbilicus. Miss Scarfe became hysterical, called him a screaming Dervish and demonstrated a command of explicit vocabulary surprising in an elderly spinster. Fortunately, I don’t believe Dr Qasimayya understood any of it, but I suspect he got the drift. Unfortunately, Miss Scarfe has not let anyone near her since including my nurses so something will have to be done”.

Everyone looked at one another, the two steel blue eyes moved from left to right and back again strafing the lot of them, even Freddie flinched.

The Pharaoh pointed both his arms to the ceiling and then thrust them apart in a gesture of despair or perhaps it was prayer, while mumbling something incomprehensible to the assembled gathering.

“See, see, he’s gibbering, what did I tell you, off his trolley he is, I came in to be cured and all I get is attacked by a mad Gippo and stared at by a bunch of darkies.”

Vera lapsed back onto her pillow; the sickness and the pain began to cloud her up-till-then clear eyes. Freddie the compassionate humourist saw his chance and adopted his Peter Sellars Indian dialect imitation and spoke with exaggerated formality to this prickly but frightened Geordie great aunt.

“My good white woman, I am the son of a chief, mine is a fierce warlike tribe, we are cannibals too.” He paused for effect; Vera’s pupils dilated a little. “We enjoy eating white men, cooking them slowly in hot stones, but the greatest delicacy is the white woman.” He leaned forward quickly, and Vera shut her eyes. “So tender, so delicate, so aromatic.

It is the meat from the palm of the hand that is the sweetest. Ah the memories of those good dinners come flooding back to me". Freddie was holding the old lady's hand now and smiled at her. There was a long silence, Vera slowly opened her eyes and stared at the Afghan Prince, and then she smiled.

"Eeeh you're havin' me on." She looked hard at Freddie to be sure, he just continued smiling. "Perhaps yer alreet after all, me nephew said you were a good un, if it's you to do it gan on, dee what you have to dee and lets be done with it." She let go of the sheet and was a model patient from then on. The operation to remove a large colonic polyp was a success and she cheated the great reaper again, but she would not let the Pharaoh near her.

She did have to stay in the hospital some weeks and her already run-down bungalow assumed an air of dereliction and neglect. The evening of her discharge some local youths decided it looked a good bet for a spot of pillage and vandalism.

It was round about eleven at night when they broke in, the mustiness and the cold confirmed their belief that the place was empty, so they made no attempt to be quiet. Vera was awakened from her light post hospital slumber by the sound of these three lads rummaging about in the Ottoman trunk at the end of her bed.

She was ever a courageous old bird and she sat bolt upright in the moonlit gloom. No wig on so no hair, no teeth and in a shroud like old lace nighty, she yelled at her burglars in a high-pitched crackly voice; "So what do ye lot think you're doin'? Gerrout or I'll set the dogs on ye all." The fact that she had never owned more than a Pekinese in her whole life was of little interest to the terrified marauders.

This ghastly spectre so unnerved them that they fled as if all the hounds of Hell were biting at their heels. I doubt they ever continued with a life of crime, though possibly one of them, haunted by such a vision in his formative years, became a Video producer for Michael Jackson.

Back at the Ranch an uneasy truce prevailed, the open hostility had gone but the tension was palpable, mealtimes were especially difficult. The two staff were determined to improve this state of affairs.

The main entrance to the Doctors' quarters was via a cluttered old Victorian style kitchen, full of hanging pots, boiled cabbage smell, large knives with ground down blades and unidentifiable bubbling concoctions on various gas rings.
The staff consisted of Madge the Cook and Ena the everything else. Madge was short and round, she had a figure like a prehistoric fertility goddess and an outrageous opinion on any topic. She seemed to live at the ranch, although she had a family of six teenagers she never seemed to go home.
Neither did Ena, who was a tall, out of a bottle blond, who always wore very red lipstick and lots of mascara, like Madge she was probably about 45 but it was not easy to know, she was childless but apparently happily married to a husband no one ever saw. The two of them never stopped talking, arguing often shouting, it was like the Duchess and the Cook in Alice but with the roles reversed.
Madge, like most on South Tyneside, was a rabid socialist by declaration but with such right-wing views as to make the then topical Enoch Powell look moderate.
She loved goading the foreign doctors with downright racist remarks, delivered in a rumbustious take that and lump it style that made any limp liberal unused to her behaviour wince with pain and embarrassment, though Madge saw herself as a gentle tease with a heart of gold.
Ena was the appeaser who would try to excuse Madge's more outrageous utterings and tone down her milder jibes with soothing excuses to the audience, which of course only stimulated Madge to go one better. The whole dialogue usually took place in amongst the steam and strange cooking smells where figures could appear and disappear in a quite eerie fashion where the grin of the Cheshire cat would not have seemed incongruous.
For their part the insulted Doctors, as a defence mechanism, began to try to exchange banter in kind, so conversations usually took the form of mutually escalating insults frequently interrupted by Ena's high pitched:
"Eeeh you mustna say that that's aawful." Madge for all her vitriol was essentially good humoured and most exchanges ended in laughter plus a final stinging Parthian shot from the steamy mist.
The mixed religions of the Subcontinent were ignored entirely by Madge in her menu construction.

She cooked an unending sequence of dumplings, steak and kidney pie and pudding, stewed cabbage and corned beef fritters with mashed potato followed by treacle tart or semolina pudding. She never seemed to notice or care that this fare was less than rapturously received; it was good enough for her own men folk, so it was good enough for the foreigners.

Freddie saw his tale telling stratagem was losing its effectiveness and decided that perhaps an attack on the menu would be a powerful unifying force.

By remarks here and there over a period of a week or so he managed to foment a reasonably good natured revolution and the opposing camps drew together in condemnation of the uninspiring diet foisted upon them, gradually the temperature of the exchanges rose.

"Hey Madge, what about a decent curry?"

"Why, that's nasty hot stuff, ruins good meat, only daft foreigners would eat that muck."

"Eeeh you mustna say that."

"Well, I say warra I mean, youse lot are in England now and you should eat wor fud, when in Rome they say."

"Yes, Madge but we are not in Rome, a pizza or a spaghetti Bolognese would be good, but a curry would be best. We would even cook it ourselves."

"Over my dead body, none of youse lot is setting a paw in my kitchen." Madge looked defiantly at the seated doctors with plates of only slightly nibbled corn beef fritters and sensed a tide she had not experienced before, a feeling of genuine rebellion, Ena broke the deadlock.

"Aw gan on Madge, you show em, make em a Madge special curry."

"Yes, go on Madge make us a special curry, cheer us all up."

Madge made her mind up, "OK Hinnies, I'll show you buggers what a curry should really be like.

I'll bet I can make a canny curry, better than any of youse lot. Ye better put the bog roll in fridge now because you'll need it."

Having picked up the gauntlet she was determined to put on a good show, and even more determined to show her Doctors that she really was a cosmopolitan cook and that the regular fritters were due to economics and not to lack of inspiration or skill.

(Or to the fact that half the Doctor's budget was probably siphoned off to feed her own family.)

She rummaged through her cupboards, and raided the main hospital stores for any spices, raisins lentils and rice that could be found. One morning the Pharaoh met her coming to work with a large brown paper parcel and a smile of defiant satisfaction on her face. She beamed at him and patted her parcel; "Abdulla from Chi's best hot curry powder, all the chillies in the East in this stuff, blow the arse off that Sphinx of yours, guaranteed five star bum burner." The Pharaoh smiled at her uncomprehendingly and offered "You soon to make good curry, I look it forward, you best cook Madge."

As you may already have gathered Madge suffered from the widespread Northern delusion that for a curry to be any good it had to lift off the top of the head while simultaneously shrivelling the tonsils, subtle nuances of flavour were not for her, this was heroic cookery.

At last, the great day dawned; Ena had prepared the dining room with a finicky thoroughness. The tables were all pushed together to make a square and the best tablecloth was produced from some hidden store.

Ena had even found 10 sets of chopsticks and set them on the table under the mistaken impression that they were the traditional implements for curry eating purposes, she also thoughtfully provided spoons and forks for the less culturally aware.

She even put flowers in the centre of the table, the get well soon message in the middle of them betraying their origins. Ena had also gone to the trouble of writing the Doctor's names on little cards and had made sure of an even mix of the warring factions. She had run out of these by the time she got to the Pharaoh and he had a bigger card with FAIRO on one side and Pathology Request on the other.

Ena summoned the doctors to their places wearing a tight fitting blue Crimplene short-skirted dress and a little frilly edged white pinafore. She wore even more lipstick and mascara than usual. The doctors filed in and found their place setting; some tried to swap to be next to an ally, but Ena was having none of it.

"You stay where you're put, this is Madge and mine's treat and you'll do it wor way or there's no dinner for ye, right?"

Sheepishly the Doctors bowed to a superior force and sat down to try to make the best of it.

Madge resplendent in a large chef's hat and for once a clean white starched smock strutted into the room bearing a tray of various side dishes; cucumber raita, vegetable curry and a spinach Bhaji, ground coconut, raisins and a large jar of pickled eggs. This latter dish is a strange Northern delicacy; usually consumed with copious quantities of Newcastle Brown Ale, a heavy deep brown beer known locally then as 'Journey into Space'. The beer is required to wash away the disgusting bitter vinegar taste, as a guide to the uninitiated the nearest experience to eating a pickled egg is probably chewing a freshly painted old tennis ball. Madge thought they were so disgusting that the foreign Doctors were sure to love them.

Ena brought in a large salver covered in steaming speckled Pilaw rice and gingerly pushed it to the centre of the table dangerously exposing a large area of heavily veined white thigh and a set of suspenders usually only seen in Sunday paper adverts. Freddie's hand approached the forbidden zone and Ena automatically brushed it away as if shooing an annoying little fly.

Then came Madge struggling with a largish black Shakespearean cauldron three quarters full of a powerful smelling, bubbling lumpy brown mixture which she triumphantly placed on the table. She stood short squat, with her ample bosomed chest stuck out challenging the assembled company to share her culinary achievement.

"Right lads this is Madge's special lamb curry," she half bowed and flourished her chef's hat like a medieval courtier, "get yer gobs roond that little lot and a diven't want any moanin'."

Ena and Madge set about helping to dispense generous helpings all round and then retired to one side of the room to await the unstinting praise that would surely follow. The luckless smiling Pharaoh was the first to try a large undiluted mouthful of the dark dripping meat. He chewed and swallowed it quickly, gesturing at Madge and Ena with an Anglicised thumbs up sign, but at that moment a change came upon him.

His normally dark and swarthy complexion suddenly changed to the same colour as the nicotine stained white wallpaper, but in another instant, there was another chameleon like change to a deep bluish green hue and within a few more seconds his whole face became a sort of reddish black.

Everyone in the room was transfixed by this 'son et Lumiere' virtuoso performance. Suddenly a choking agonised deep Egyptian oath escaped from his lips and echoed eerily round the room. He shot bolt upright, knocking his chair over in the process, clutched his throat and ran, wild eyed, from the room.

This happening had a somewhat unnerving effect on the spectators. Complete silence engulfed the table, fatty brown lumps were pushed gingerly around plates, lumps were dissected into tiny pieces smothered in rice and chewed with extreme nervous deliberation whilst anxiously watching the others for signs of acute toxicity. In fact, after the first two or three mouthfuls the pain went, to be replaced by a buzzing numb feeling extending from the forehead to the Adam's apple.

The experience even became pleasurable in a masochistic sort of way. Madge, somewhat disconcerted by the Pharaoh's exit, ventured a prompt.

"Well, worra ye think then?"

Those who could speak were mainly from Southern India, used to fearsomely hot curries.

"Bit much chilli Madge but not bad for a Memsahib." Others nodded as best they could and gradually the curry and the side dishes began to disappear, conversation returned, even became animated and sworn enemies laughed together. Briefly the mess was a happy place. After a while Madge voiced the anxiety of the others;

"Where's that fond fool the Pharaoh, aah think a bit must've gone doon the wrang way if ye ask me. Ena be a gud lass an gan and luk fer him, make sure he's alreet."

Ena found him some time later clutching the children's drinking fountain in the hospital car park, with a deathly pale complexion, streaming eyes and an absolute inability to speak. She led him back to his room like a sick animal and stayed with him some time. He never ate in the mess again. Only existing on a diet of Egyptian biscuits sent from home, salami sausage and rye bread from a grocer over the road, but Ena went to his room a lot after that day, her suspendered thighs offering him some solace in a lonely country.

Not long afterwards a curry house opened opposite the hospital ambitiously titled "The Gourmet", this was too much for the Geordie tongue and it was soon universally known as "The Gummit".

Once a week the doctors clubbed together and enjoyed a glutinous take away evening. Madge was never called on to perform again but was held in increased respect by the entire mess from the time of that memorable meal.
As for the Pharaoh, with Ena's help, he struggled through the last few months of his attachment, doctors and nurses alike seeing to it that he was as far as possible kept away from any patients, especially sick ones. He gave up his English lessons but took up painting; he was actually very good at it. Just before he left, he presented the mess with a large canvas of the famous curry evening; he called it "The Last Supper".

Mickey, Sunderland General, February 1969
Sunderland General outpatient's department in February 1969 was not the most fun filled place to be. I don't need to describe it your imagination will do better, but I warn you, it was worse than that. It is shut now; it had been the old workhouse (as had South Shields General) and was a deeply depressing and forbidding building.
I was the medical house officer drafted in to see the 'chronics'. These were the living dead, with advanced incurable illnesses that medicine had no solution for, and precious little comfort. As the most junior doctor in the hospital, it was reasoned I couldn't make them any worse and the cleverer doctors could be utilised on the newer patients who might just be more interesting if no less curable. It was late in the afternoon, I was subdued, a little cowed by the inevitability of it all, remember I was only 22 and wanted to make a difference to peoples' suffering but there didn't seem to be a way. Then I met Mickey.
He was a little man, maybe five foot nothing in his socks, a chest like a barrel and a cherubic pink face with a smile to make your heart ache. He struggled into the cubicle, room would be too posh a word, gasping and clutching from one support to another. He was looking at me the whole time. He spoke in gasps that didn't seem to have any pauses between them. He had a chirrupy cheeky voice.
'Way Hinney, yor not oot of school surely, and yer the wrang colour fer this place. Ye need a coat of broon paint to be a doctor in Sunland.' I was on my feet trying to help him, he shooed me away.
'Divvent need any help, be in me box soon enough, aal gerrall the help then, that's what the Vicar says, but he's run off with the missus, so what would he kna, poor bugger.'

He cackled wheezily, and sat with a rush, panting. I thought he was going to die there and then. I had no idea what I was supposed to do for Mickey, but this was not a unique feeling that afternoon. Mickey took a minute or so to get what little was left of his breath back; I saw he was dressed in his Sunday best. Collar, tie, starched shirt, full suit with waistcoat and silver fob chain and shiny black brogues. He looked like he had just been redeemed from the pawnshop. He smelt overpoweringly of Vick and mothballs. In extremis there are standards to be maintained, he was doing that. Many of these attitudes died with his generation and we are the poorer for it. But Mickey was the most fearlessly irreverent of men.

'Wey gan on, ask me how I am, do they teach you nuthin these days?'

'Er how are you Mr Scott?' I obeyed, knowing I was outranked. Here was a dying man with experience of living, it was his show.

'Bloody knackered, aav nor enuff puff to blow oot a Lucifer.' He was triumphant to have got his opening gambit out with a finality that left few avenues to explore. I couldn't think of anything to say. I vaguely remembered that Lucifer was First World War slang for match, some expressions linger in little communities.

'Lucifer, that's an odd word, match isn't it?'

He broke into wheezy song 'While you've a Lucifer to light your fag, smile boys that's the style, pack up your troubles in your old kit bag and smile smile smile.' He regrouped. 'Sang that at Dunkirk, drooned the noise of them Jerry Bastards in the Stukas. Me Da must have sung it too.

Go to Wipers an put yer ear to the groond on Hill 16 and you might hear him singing it, a hundred feet doon.' I waited as he left no gap for me to enter into. 'He was a miner too, didn't live lang enough to die slow like me, boom and half of bloody Belgium on top of him. Aah were 3 months at the time.' I felt I ought to be a doctor not a listener, always an unwise move, so I butted in.

'Do you need a new inhaler?'

He looked at me with a sort of head shaking smile of despair for the ignorant. 'Look yer daft happorth, yam tryin me best to tell you me story an your gannin on aboot puffers. Look young doc let's be clear. You can't cure me, aah doot you can help me but the least ye can do is listen to me. Aave cum in me best canonicals, an its norraneasy journey from Hetton. Give me some respect an I meet larn you summat.'

‘Like what?’ I said a trifle crossly, it was late, I was nearly but not quite fed up and Mickey was the last patient that afternoon.
‘Aboot what it’s like to be poorly. Ifn yer gannin to be any gud you’ve gorra understand what yer patients are gannin thru. De yees kna with the help of me missus, she didna run off with the vicar more’s the pity, it took we nearly an hour just to get togged up to gan oot.
We had to keep stoppin just to get breath. She had to put me troosers on us for God’s sake. You imagine that young un?’ I didn’t want to, I was unsure where this was leading but I have always liked stories, it seemed there were worse things to do than listen to Mickey’s. I hadn’t learned the trick of saying ‘tell me more’ but Mickey was going to tell me whether I liked it or not. He looked into my eyes, right in deep, much deeper than any examiner I had met.
‘Ye kna anythin aboot mining? Aave been doon Hetton pit since I were 14 with fower years off for gud behaviour scrappin with the Hun. An yer kna why aam like I am, its cos ạave got a bag of nutty slack in me chest.’ I obviously looked confused.
‘Nutty slack is them crappy little bits of coal they canna sell so the pit owners generously hand it oot free to the workers, but if you’ve been doon lang enough you’ve already got a sackful in yer chest. Ifn yer set fire to us aad born for a week. You want ter see me spit.’ It wasn’t a question. Mickey took out a tightly wrapped little pot from an inside pocket.
Sputum is not a glamorous human secretion, but this was different, the now unwrapped pot was opened to reveal a slimy translucent substance full of tiny black bits, there could be no doubt these little bits were indeed coal. An image of dissected black lungs shown in some long nearly forgotten previous lecture came to mind, I knew now quite clearly what Mickey’s lungs looked like from the inside, I felt a wave of sympathy, he saw it.
‘Aah don’t want yer pity but now ye kna what aam talkin aboot. There’s none of yer medicines can get rid of that lot, ye kna the worst? Me missus is forever buyin washin pooder cos me hankies is allas (always) black with hoiking (coughing) this stuff into them.’
He cackled again, I still didn’t know if he wanted anything of me, but whatever it was it was not sympathy.

'You a local lad?' I nodded. 'Like football?' I nodded again.
'Sunland?' I kept nodding 'Charley Horley (Hurley)?' I smiled a big smile. Big Charlie was and remains my all-time Sunderland hero, a magnificent attacking centre half and a leader of men.
'Dooin rotten at present mind you.' This was sadly true, nothing changes. 'Not won a game al year, ye kna my favourite? Captain Raich (Carter), Shack was pretty canny (Len Shackleton) but the Captain, he was summit special.
Aah canna gan anymore, didna miss a match for 30 yors but aah haven't the puff now, aah canna gerrup the stairs. Shame but at least I tell mesel there's nowt worth watchin. Dee yer want to listen?'
'Listen?'
'To me chest! they all want to listen, though gawd knas what fower. Howay give us a hand wi me jacket and we'll find a gap fer yer tubes.'
We did after a struggle. Mickey breathed and I listened. I expected wheezing and rattling but could not hear anything.
I checked my stethoscope. Mickey grinned triumphantly. 'Nowt to hear eh, one of them top clever clogs showed me off to the students once. Mister Taylor,' he said in an exaggeratedly posh voice, 'has no sounds in his lungs because he has no air in them, you need air to produce the sound, he has silent lungs, a very advanced sign I am afraid.'
He slipped back into deepest Wearside. 'That were five years ago an he's deed, heart attack, an aam still battin. He said aah was a pink puffer. Aah thowt he was talkin aboot a train but when he said the other sort was a blue bloater ah thowt he'd been doon to the fish quay. But ye kna, a couple of me mates were big an' blue all ower, they're in their boxes noo.' Mickey was referring to the traditional description of the two types of respiratory failure, usually seen in miners.
Skinny small gasping men who stayed pink to the end and their friends who developed heart strain and then heart failure, known by the Latin name of Cor Pulmonale. They filled up with fluid and were cyanosed all of the time because not enough oxygen got into their blood stream to make it the usual red colour. I began to help him get his jacket back on and mentioned the possibility of a flu injection.

'Hadaway there's na point, de ye think ah want to keep living like this? Aah want the reaper to come, sooner the better if ye ask me, protect us from flu!! It would be a god's blessing to get a quick vicious one kidda. The day I have one of them jabs will be the day I snuff it.' Prophetic as it turned out. 'I betta be away noo, divvent want to miss the bus and ye've had enough for one day.'

'I haven't done anything for you.'

'Nor you have kidda, but you've been a change. 3 months if I'm still here?'

It was only the next week that Mickey ended up in the medical ward; he was grey and in extremis but still joking.

"You still here?" he said recognising me "Aah thowt you'd be back in kindergarten."

I wish someone would say that to me today.

Little Mackem miners did not die easily, however. He struggled on for a few weeks, wearing a sort of nighty as he hated anything tight, at night he also wore a bed cap, sister christened him 'Wee Willy Winky': he needed virtually continuous oxygen provided by an array of heavy black cylinders surrounding his bed; Mickey said it felt like being in a U Boat.

At night you could spot Mickey's cot by the bright glow of his woodbine, burning beautifully in almost pure oxygen. No one stopped him, they had grown to love him too much besides all the nurses smoked in those days, as did I; in fact, a communal name for nurses on night duty was a fug.

Mickey's spirit remained uncrushed by illness and the haunted look of the dying was conspicuously absent, there was no reproach in his eyes. The only time I saw fear was shortly before he died, I was hurrying through my examination that day and he spotted it "Where's the fire Doc?"

I told him it was my job to immunise all the hospital staff against Hong Kong flu that day and that I was already late.

"Well, aam dyin' and there is nowt to do but keep me comfy so gan on and keep the livin' healthy, aam a bit fed up mind you so if aam still around toneet promise you'll give me one them jabs you're givin'." It seemed an odd logic but who was I to argue. I was about to go when he caught my hand and held it.

"Promise me Doc." There was a brief glimpse of real fear deep in those black eyes "you won't let them bury me, will you?

I will make a good fire, but I couldn't stand all that earth on me for eternity, aave been under the ground too lang already. The missus wants me next to her lot on Hetton Hill but Aah want me ashes on Roker Park. Promise me." So, I did.
We were too efficient at immunising as it turned out; we did all the staff in one frenetic day. But the vaccine was a rush job and improperly centrifuged, so It was the next day when 75% of the nurses and doctors did not turn up for work because of reactions to the jab that caused the crisis. Mickey joshed that as there was no one to look after him it was time he went; he insisted on the flu jab and held my hand.
"A promise is a promise." I nodded; he relaxed and died peacefully that night. His wife in fact told me she would never bury him as she understood his fear and promised to get one of his sons to take his ashes to the football ground. They did win the next home game. I did not have a flu jab for 40 years till my new wife insisted. They don't make them like Mickey anymore.

The Royal Northern Hospital Holloway Rd
It was February 1970, and I was having an interview for a job in a posh consulting room in Harley Street. At this stage I had finished my house jobs and had a six month spell in Australia on a P&O liner.
It was time to see if London's streets were in fact paved with gold. They certainly were in Harley Street. My interview was with a slightly cross Scottish surgeon and obstetrician who had his Rolls Royce pointedly parked right outside the door.
He only asked me 2 questions, when I could start and was I any good at stitching?
I asked him where the hospital was, and he said that finding it was a condition of employment. I worked at the hospital for nine months, looked after his private patients but never set eyes on him again. The hospital in question was the Royal Northern Hospital, Holloway Rd, now closed.
A small hospital founded 100 years or so earlier by an aggrieved surgeon called Statham who had been suspended from UCH for slapping a lady patient's bottom!
I had just been appointed a casualty officer but within a week I found I was also the ENT SHO, the obstetric SHO for private patients and once a week acting medical registrar on call.

This suited me fine, experience was what I was after. I had no girlfriend at the time and for the first four weeks never left the hospital and was always on duty. It was a very busy little casualty department and looked down on literally and metaphorically by its sister department at the Whittington.

By the end of this month, I found myself chairman/treasurer of the doctor's bar, being a Geordie the Londoners thought that this was a natural appointment. To my horror I found there was a strange system of writing the drinks orders in an A four book with the prices, and then payment was by bill at the end of each month.

The problem of course was that by the time several drinks had been consumed and doctor's writing being appalling at the best of times, the later entries were completely illegible. I asked a friend what previous bar chairmen had done. He shrugged and said that if he was me, he would add up the total monthly bill and divide it by the number of doctors in the hospital and send everyone a bill. I said that that was a ridiculous idea and that many of the doctors were of course teetotal, again he shrugged and said just try it, so I did. Amazingly 95% of the doctors just paid up including teetotal ones and the recovered bar receipts were up by 50%. This was true communism in action.

It was a fairly small hospital of around 200 beds and 20 private beds, the chief surgeon was Reg Murley, then president of the RCS, an inspiring if somewhat daunting character.

The chief physician was Gerry James, the Sarcoid king, whose even more famous wife was Sheila Sherlock, the doyenne of hepatology, and a close mentor of our very own Howard Thomas (with whom I shared a corpse in 63/4 and now live nearby) who went on to be professor of medicine at Imperial specialising in livers.

My most dramatic recollection of Sheila was when playing cricket against the Whittington hospital in front of that huge gothic mental asylum, Friern Barnet.

She was umpiring, a small figure covered in sweaters and hats, and while in a dramatic partnership with the aforesaid Reg Murley gave me out lbw to a ball missing the leg stump by at least a yard, well that's my story anyway.

In those days London was easier to travel across and my favourite pub was the Waterman's Arms on the Isle of Dogs, now also gone. When you got there a bunch of Millwall urchins always approached.

"Mind your car sir?" It was a foolish customer that didn't give them half a crown. I had a brief liaison with a final year medical student from the Royal Free hospital and one night the local Chas and Dave type combo were raising the roof with old cockney songs. The Pearly Kings and Queens were there in full regalia too when my companion asked the barman for a set of spoons and proceeded to demonstrate a remarkable talent. She was a full figured girl and her ability to play the spoons off the more dramatic pieces of her anatomy brought the house down. I didn't buy a drink that night.

The Berge Istra.

It is May 1972, and I am senior surgeon on the one class P&O liner SS Orcades. This voyage has lasted for six months and it is time to go home. Perth is a pretty city, my daughter lives there now, Fremantle, its port, was not then. So, there was little regret on our departure as we set off across the wide expanse of the Indian Ocean; our next landfall, Durban, being five full sailing days away with no land in sight at all till then. It was the longest single stretch Orcades ever sailed; this was puny however to the route currently being taken by the ship that was soon to play such a dramatic part in our lives. 24 hours out of Fremantle I was awoken by the 2nd Sparks (Radio Officer) telling me I was wanted in the Radio Room for an urgent medical consultation with an unnamed ship's master.

This experience was not entirely infrequent; only passenger ships and naval vessels carried doctors and it was maritime convention that all other ships could call up the nearest ship with a doctor for advice. This was of course long before the internet, satellite phones and the like. As a young medic I was used to being roused from sleep, performing some medical function, and going quickly back to sleep and still being fresh as a daisy the next day. It is only past 40 that this facility wanes.

I was quite chipper despite it being 2 am and it was not a long walk, you could see the radio room from my cabin door.

I was handed the chunky radio telephone, the reception, as ever, was poor, much crackling and hissing and a nervous voice speaking rapidly in poor English with a thick Scandinavian accent. I got the drift that there had been an accident and that a senior crew member was seriously injured, but how seriously?

The line went down and was then restored, the reception was a little improved and I was getting my ear in.

The Master, for it was he on the phone, repeated the story. It was his Chief Electrician who had been repairing electrical wiring on top of one of the ship's boilers, he had received a severe shock (the ship worked on 480 volts) and had been catapulted backwards and fallen at least 20 feet. He was still alive, but the Captain feared he was dying and needed more assistance than he and his crew could provide.

The company, P&O, that was my employer, did not mind me dispensing medical advice to all and sundry; they did mind if it altered the Ship's itinerary because that cost money.

So, the onus was on the Surgeon to deal with medical matters there and then with whatever advice that seemed useful and avoid at all costs any rendezvous unless it really was a matter of life and death, and even then, you had to be as sure as possible that the patient would live with your ministrations and die without them. If he was going to die anyway that was just hard luck. This meant I had to become a medical interrogator, to glean as many facts as possible and to get as clear a risk benefit profile as possible, in order to make the difficult decision whether to suggest intervention or not. The ultimate decision was not mine to take, that was the Captain's, and he would usually consult with the company.

After a series of very direct questions to the Master and then to the 2nd mate, who was acting as the medic and who's English was better, I began to get a clearer picture of what injuries the electrician had sustained. Firstly, he was in a lot of pain, so ascertaining his weight I gave advice on the appropriate dose and frequency of morphine that the ship was carrying in its medical supplies. The nature of the pain suggested chest wall injuries, front and back, and possible vertebral damage in the lower thoracic and upper lumbar region.

Fortunately, there was apparently no sign of paralysis so for the moment it did not seem that the spinal cord had been damaged, though if there was a fractured vertebra injudicious movement could be disastrous. The two most pressing worries were that he was peeing blood and getting paler and iller by the hour. This strongly suggested internal injury to at least one kidney and possible internal bleeding due to injury to other organs such as the liver or spleen.

If, as seemed likely, he had several fractured ribs the displaced jagged ends could easily spear such organs, with very unpleasant consequences.

The most unpleasant of which was dying of internal haemorrhage. This poor man was in deep trouble, but could we help him? I gave what advice I could on fluid intake, care with moving him, and monitoring of his condition, such as pulse and blood pressure which fortunately the 2nd mate had been trained to take; then arranged to take bulletins 2 hourly. In the meanwhile, I promised to discuss rendezvous with my Captain.

He was not best pleased at being woken in the middle of the night; he was well past 40.

He was also perturbed; this was a bad time to have to consider slowing down as there were a whole array of deadlines ahead and it being such a long crossing fuel as well as being costly was also in limited supply. Stopping and restarting engines apparently used up a disproportionate amount of the stuff. He was a good man though with a humanitarian soul, he wanted to do what was right, but he had to be sure. I was to report back after the next medical bulletin but in the meanwhile the Officer of the Watch was to ascertain the speed and direction of the other ship and work out the most efficient course needed to converge, with the implicit baseline that if there was any major alteration of course needed this was to be up to the other ship. The two hours passed in no time and the report indicated that he was probably worsening. His blood pressure seemed to be slipping downwards as his pulse rose, a bad combination and further indication of likely internal bleeding. He probably needed surgery and he would soon definitely need blood, both ships were a minimum of 2 days from land in any direction. There is a commonly held myth that anything serious that goes wrong on a ship can be rectified by dispatching a helicopter, this is rubbish even now and it was certainly rubbish in 1972.

The range for a helicopter is quite small, with only 2-3 hours sailing most ships were out of range unless hugging the coast.

We were by now nearly 48 hours away from Australia, way out of range of any such aid.

In the meanwhile, the company had made it plain to our Captain that there was to be no turning back as part of any equation. He told me this as he weighed the options, he appreciated that it was my medical recommendation that the electrician should be taken on board to give him at least a fighting chance.

We could probably transfuse him and in desperation even operate as he was, he was likely to die in the next day or so.

We had found out the name of the ship, she was called the Berge Istra, but our Lloyds list did not have information on her. Presumably she was too new. Remember the internet was still a long time in the future. We also knew her course now, she was on what was termed 'a grand circle' from Buenos Arias to Yokohama, an enormous distance to cover without stopping; you need to look at globe to understand where we were intersecting.
Her Master had agreed to alter course and ours had been given permission to stop for as short a period as possible to take the ill man on board. We were going to meet in about 12 hours. We all hoped, but for many different reasons, that it would not be too late.
The Captain invited me to the Bridge to get the first glimpse of the Berge Istra. The recent medical reports on the electrician were worrying but he was still alive. At last, the Bosun shouted and pointed to a blip on the Radar, we stared at it. The Captain squinted, 'That's a flaming big blip!' He exclaimed and looked with binoculars at the horizon; he shook his head in disbelief as he handed them to me.
'The size of her Surgeon, just look at the size of her!'

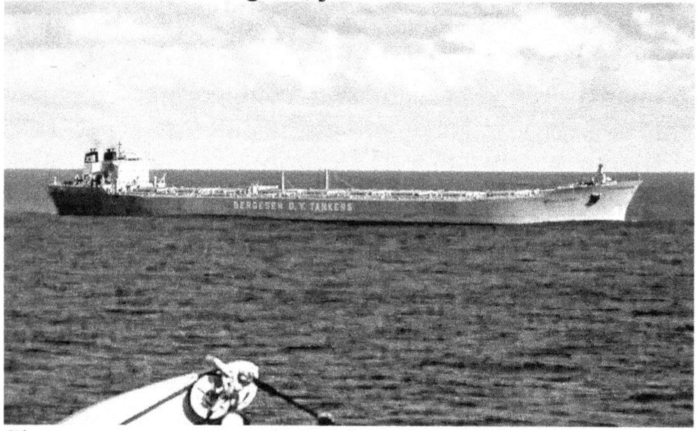

She was a monster, a huge, long green monster. As she came alongside our relative sizes became plain.
We were a big passenger ship for the time, 28,000 tons give or take, but we could have been a lifeboat for this one; it transpired that at that moment she was the biggest ship on the planet.
Both ships stopped alongside but at some distance, there was a big swell running, and we were still about a quarter of a mile away, as close as both Captains dared.

She was a colossal multipurpose carrier and brand spanking new, her very size calmed the sea between the two vessels.
She was twin funnelled positioned as far aft as possible behind the slab like Bridge and living quarters, in front of the quarters was a huge stretch of deck with at least 9 large battened down hatches. Emblazoned in large white letters against the green sides was the inscription, Bergesen D.Y. Tankers. I knew I should go over to her to supervise the bringing over of the injured man, but our Captain refused to let me go.
He said it was too risky and he couldn't afford to lose a surgeon, but I suspected it was because it would take too much time. It was a big disappointment. The passengers were all crowding the upper decks to marvel at this leviathan and watch the show, the word was out that we were picking up a severely injured sailor. It was too great a distance to attach a line between the two ships, but they were great professionals that crew of the Berge Istra.
In an amazingly short time, they had lowered a tiny looking little red lifeboat, strapped the injured man into a wraparound stretcher, named after its designer, Anderson, and secured him as tightly as possible. The lifeboat bobbed across in double quick time. We had opened the aft door, to be nearer the hospital, and the lifeboat docked; seven large sailors gently but quickly unloaded their comrade. They shook hands, accepted a crate of whiskey with our Captain's compliments and were off again. The whole transfer took less than 20 minutes. Both ships restarted engines, hooted at each other, the passengers cheered and the Berge Istra's amazingly small crew waved back, and we went our separate ways, but the memory of that great green beauty is still vivid, nearly 50 years later. I can see it now.
We had our patient on board and carried him to the hospital when the first problem presented itself. He, like his ship, was huge. So huge that he was too long for our hospital beds, he was 6ft 8in tall. We made him comfortable on one bed while the Ship's Carpenter sawed off the foot of the other bed.
He was pale as a ghost, but able to talk and his English was good though his nationality was Swedish. His name was Hans, and he was very poorly.
His pulse was thin and fast, his blood pressure low and he was in agony every time he urinated because of blood clots in the pee.

On closer examination it seemed that a lower left rib had ripped into the left kidney, more ominously it looked like he had a ruptured spleen too. His abdomen was tense, exquisitely tender and the muscle hardened on light touch, a medical sign of internal inflammation known as guarding.

This was probably due to blood in the peritoneal cavity but could indicate a ruptured bowel. If that was the case, he was definitely a goner. All in all, his chances of reaching Durban did not look too bright, and the first priority was to give him some blood and keep his pain as controlled as possible.

This was not easy at this time on a passenger liner, we could not carry stores of blood, and the blood substitutes available then were not much good. The cross matching was primitive, done with a series of blotting papers, a methodology devised by a Norwegian, which did in the end save a Swede from a Norwegian ship. I had a list of blood groups of crew who were prepared to donate blood in emergency.

I cross matched Hans and again luck was not on his side. It was not on Colin's side either. Colin was the Chief Officer, and the only person listed that was AB+ like Hans. He was a big florid man, but he was a lot less florid by the time we got to Durban. In fact, when I asked him to come to the hospital and it gradually became clear to him that he was only person that stood between this huge Swede and eternity all the colour drained out of his cheeks and his normal ebullient expansiveness evaporated, but he knew his duty. We hitched Colin up to the bottle, with those old red rubber tubes now long since replaced by transparent plastic, and took a pint off him, which we gave straight to Hans. It was for such a big man a drop in a bucket, but we gave him some reconstituted plasma to bulk it out too. After a few hours the clot colic began easing and his urine began to clear, so at least the kidney bleeding was stopping, but what about the spleen?

Operating on a passenger liner at this time was very much a last resort.

Putting people to sleep is easy, well in our case easyish; the trick is waking them up again and not gassing yourself in the process.

This meant that our strategy had to be to avoid operation if humanly possible and to try to keep poor Hans alive for the 3 more days to Durban, but if operation was his only chance…. I got out the surgical textbooks.

Human beings, unlike cars or washing machines, do not come with detailed repair manuals, more's the pity. The nearest we had then were surgical and anatomical textbooks. I read the bit on spleens, cut along dotted line A, tie off B, dissect out C etc, poor Hans, he hadn't got a hope. An appendix I could just about manage but a splenectomy, no way.
I phoned Colin again, how was he feeling? He got the drift immediately; you did not need a videophone to visual his expression. He bravely 'volunteered' to donate another pint.
I can't take all of the credit for this noble self-sacrifice; it was really down to Brenda the nurse, who at this time was having a brief but extremely physical relationship with the aforesaid Colin. That was if the noises emanating out of her cabin late at night were to be taken at face value.
I have reason to believe that to stiffen, if that is the right word, Colin's shaky resolve the spirit of the Greek Play Lycistrita was invoked.
You will remember that this was a group of women who withdrew conjugal favours from their men till they bucked their ideas up and went to war.
After the second pint Hans really did start to improve. His blood pressure stabilised, his pulse rate at last started dropping below a hundred, his temperature was down, and, perhaps most importantly, he began to think he might make it. He began chatting, and Brenda took his personal details down. He was born in Gothenburg, but his current domicile was an address in the Scotty Road Liverpool where he was ensconced with a Scouser young lady. He had met the Beatles, been regularly to the Cavern Club, and had a few drinks with John Lennon.
He had started his career aged 17 apprenticed to The Blue Funnel line, which was based in Liverpool, known after its founder as 'Alfred Holt's Navy', and got this plum job on the maiden voyage of the Berge Istra, owned by a Norwegian shipping magnate. The Istra was to be part of a fleet of huge carriers with the prefix Berge.
One reason for getting the job was his proficiency in languages; he spoke at least seven, even if his English was flavoured by a not unattractive mix of Swedish and Liverpudlian dialect. In no time he was chatting Brenda up, a fact not unnoticed by the increasingly anaemic Colin, but both men were not really up to any action, it was just fun and probably aided the healing.

With 24 hours to go Hans's condition took a turn for the worse, probably because he was trying to do too much and shuffled off to the loo by himself rather than suffer the indignity and humiliation of the bed pan, the ship rolled a little, he slipped, and the bleeding started again.

I really did think we were going to have to operate this time. We gave him a large dose of morphine and a sedative to knock him out and those of a religious persuasion prayed, especially Colin.

Twelve hours to go, slow but definite deterioration, could Colin manage just a further ½ pint? He did, I don't know if he will be rewarded in heaven, but after his recovery a week or so later he was certainly rewarded on this earth according to reports. That was enough; Hans made it to Durban where the ambulance and surgical team were waiting.

He was in fact even more damaged than we had thought. Both kidneys were injured, his liver capsule was torn and oozing internally, and the spleen was ruptured.

I believe they aspirated at least 4 pints out of his peritoneal cavity. 2 and ½ of which had belonged to Colin. His spleen was removed and 1/3 of his left kidney and he was transfused a further 6 pints of blood, but he made it, and within 2 months was back in Liverpool.

For a few years he sent me Xmas Cards with little details of his life, and he was back on the Berge Istra. By this time, I was a family doctor and listening to the radio one morning while doing my visits there was a news bulletin reporting the tragic loss of one of the biggest ships in the world, yes you guessed it, the Berge Istra. She had gone down with the loss of all hands in the South China Sea.

I stopped the car and couldn't continue for some time, I just knew that Hans had not cheated death twice, Neptune would have his sacrifice. I read later that the cause was probably inadequate clearing of the holds of inflammable gasses before loading a full cargo of iron ore in Japan. There was an explosion causing a hull rupture and she had sunk like a stone. At Lloyds of London, they rang the Lutine Bell.

Her sister ship the MS Berge Vanga sank in similar circumstances four years later.

Early General Practice.

It was a Thursday in January 1974 that I was first called to visit Ethel Cramp. The message gave the reason as ‘legs.’

She lived in some council flats in the old centre of town only a few hundred yards from our Surgery. The entrance was obscure, and it took several minutes to find it. It was the lady in the health food shop who put me out of my misery.
“You the doctor come for Ethel?”
I nodded self-consciously, carrying my over large new plastic doctor’s bag and red stethoscope. She pointed to an alleyway.
“Down there, she’s on the right. Take her vitamins every week I do. Funny old trout really.”
She looked at me properly with a squinting assessment.
“You’re the new doctor? Gawd you don’t look old enough to deliver newspapers.” She smiled, “Good luck anyway.”
Ethel’s door was ajar, and a smell emanated which I did not recognise then but has become familiar to me over the years as that of human bodies past their best.
The room was dark, curtains half drawn, and there by the gas fire sat Ethel. I say sat, but this is a totally inadequate description. I don’t think there is a word in the English language to truly describes her posture. She was slumped in the chair as if she had just fallen backwards into it; her vast blue legs were apart revealing a highly inadequate gusset. Sharon Stone she wasn’t. She made an effort to focus on me, without any change in position.
“Who the fuck are you?”
I was unprepared for this greeting, stumbled over an object and became unbalanced because of my heavy, cumbersome bag, staggered dangerously towards her open crotch, stabilised myself just in time and mumbled unconvincingly.
“I am Dr Tate, the new doctor from the Ock Street Surgery.”
She looked at me with withering disbelief. I discovered an early truth then; people in their own houses had much more power than in my surgery. I was on her territory and she was boss. This was uncomfortable. There was a silence. A stale urine smell was emanating from the chair and empowered by the gas fire. My eyes started to water.
What to say? I was not in control. She gestured with frighteningly deformed hands to what seemed to be her exposed nether regions.
“Me legs.” she said.
Silence fell again. I looked at her legs more closely. Below her knees on both legs were large, ulcerated areas. The legs were massive.

She was wearing slippers but no socks. Kneeling down to get a closer look the carpet squelched, and an unnerving sensation of creeping dampness embraced my knees. My senior partner's warning came to mind too late.

"Off to see Ethel are you, well you better learn the rules quickly. In a house like hers, and there are lots, there are only two rules but never forget them or I promise you, you will regret it. Never sit down and never kneel down. Rule two, never forget the first rule."

I just had. While this unpleasant realisation was literally sinking in, my eyes, now more accustomed to the gloom could focus on the ulcers. They were huge, at least six inches across, covered in yellow foul-smelling pus, and no, surely not, there was movement.

There were maggots. A wave of nausea hit me, I gagged and fought desperately against vomiting over the urine and pus enriched carpet. That was the first visit, and all I saw then was a deformed, maggot-infested old crone who repulsed me. General practice was not going to be much fun if there were many Ethels. I was wrong, and she continued to teach me and over the months that we became accustomed to each other. Friends would be the wrong word, but Mabel thought she needed me, and I became fascinated by her story. When she was young, she loved horses. Men were incidental, and her job at the Post Office only an interruption, between the visits to the stable and the companionship of her beloved horse Elley. The day Elley died, part of Ethel died too.

She never found a replacement, drifted into marriage with an outwardly dry and inwardly shrivelled professional photographer, had two children, both girls, who gave her no pleasure, and lived an arid, joyless English life.

She was widowed at 60, both girls long gone abroad, as far from mother as they could get. Age had withered and rumpled Mabel; the bags under her eyes were spectacular, her jowls hung like a bloodhound and her chin folded like a well-used fan.

The bottom eyelids began to fold outwards in this general collapse of the flesh, giving her a doleful doggy look that was both sad and a little macabre.

By now she was heroically ugly, 16 stone with osteoarthritis of her hips and rapidly deforming hands, the knuckles swelling and the fingers falling sideways. When I met her, she had not set foot out of the door for five years. She was 72, 2 years younger than I am rewriting this recollection.

In fact, the District Nurses heroically dressed and coped with her ulcers, the Social Services department set up an efficient care package. They got her up in the morning, Meals on Wheels ('Muck in a truck' according to Ethel) fed her, the nurse assistant bed-bathed her regularly and someone came to put her to bed. My role as her doctor was very peripheral, but to her, still crucial. In her mind I was what stood between her and the grim reaper.

To me, I wasn't sure what to do, medical school hadn't really equipped me for this long-term, pastoral sort of care, but I had been taught to do things, and so I did.

I fiddled with her tablets. Someone, years ago, had diagnosed an underactive thyroid gland, and as she was always tired and sluggish, as well as being enormously overweight, I put her dose of thyroxine up to get things going. This gave me something to ask about when I visited.

"Was there any improvement?"

She teased me by offering glimmers of hope.

"A little better doctor, but my bowels are bad."

So, I gave her bowel mixture. My therapeutic courage began to rise; I experimented with diuretics to release the fluid trapped in her bloated body. Her heart was a bit irregular, so I tried digoxin, a heart stimulant, known for centuries and extracted from the foxglove plant. At last, I felt like a real doctor, I was doing something for this unfortunate old lady. By this stage she had me visiting her once a week. A ritual was developing; the care assistant left a teapot ready and two cups.

I boiled the tea, examined her while it brewed, and had a quick cup while she told me stories of the past, nearly always related to horses. The encounter would finish with me writing a new prescription for my latest experiment and telling her it was my greatest wish that one day she would be able to go to the chemist to get these herself.

After a while the ritual changed a little, and she began giving me presents. Old cameras of her husband's, tatty old Kodak box cameras.

I used to try and refuse them, but she was insistent, a level of guilt began to build up in me, and in the end, I used to pop into the Red Cross Shop across the road with each new acquisition.

Then new things were produced, hideous plastic shoehorns with antlers, tacky leather bookmarks, little chrome picture frames etc.

The guilt level rose even more, she was buying these things via an intermediary just to keep me coming regularly. Didn't she know I would come anyway, I said to myself. As the realisation of my importance to her very existence began to really impinge on my conscience, I vowed to try to do more with my professional influence. I set a goal in my mind to mobilise Ethel. To get her out of that ghastly little room for a walk in the truly fresh air.
Now every encounter finished not just with a wish but a task, to walk across the room and back, to walk into the back yard etc. She began to respond; a frame was conjured up by the nurses who also became excited by this vision of a mobile Ethel.
We professionals now aimed our whole therapeutic force into getting her to go out; it gave us a purpose. I began leading her by the hand across her sticky carpet, the presents stopped but her humour improved. A few years fell away, a light returned to the eyes; she talked of her beloved Elley.
For the first time I could actually see her, blond hair streaming, galloping across the Downs. This ruined old lady had been young, vivacious, even attractive, once.
Then came the day. A domiciliary physiotherapist had been working with her for some weeks and was convinced she was ready to try a little journey. As the physio told me this, standing in the back yard, I noticed she was clutching a large plastic shoehorn with antlers.
Mabel greeted me enthusiastically:
"I am going to bloody to do it."
She waited for a reaction; I just smiled and nodded.
"Tomorrow I'm going up the road to the naffing Post Office for me pension. Worked there for twenty year, don't suppose anyone will know me now."
She mused and continued.
"That nice girl thinks I should do it so I will."
She looked at me and I realised that I was not important anymore, that was why the presents had stopped. I should have been happy, but a little touch of pique entered my soul. It grieves me to admit it, but doctors like to be important.
The next morning, while I was seeing patients in my morning surgery, there was an emergency call. Would I go immediately to Abingdon Post Office? My patient Ethel Cramp had been involved in a serious accident; the ambulance was standing by.

All GPs hate leaving a full surgery; it ruins the day and creates a lot of tension. The story was crystal clear to me already, that Ethel had slipped off her frame, twisted her ankle or similar and that this would turn out to be a fuss about nothing. I was irritated too by the feeling that this was my own fault anyway by encouraging this unwise excursion, and naturally arrived at the scene in an unhelpful frame of mind.

There was a large crowd outside the post office where the ambulance was parked with its blue light flashing. There was another crowd about fifty yards down the road.

I parked my car behind the ambulance, waving my stethoscope at the Policeman to identify myself (a friend of mine did that once while speeding to an emergency; the policeman waved the handcuffs back).

At this time, in the early seventies, ambulance men were well-trained but not the protocol-driven, machine-like paramedics of the present day. Doctors were still required at the scene of accidents, although most doctor's training and experience in emergency medicine was none too good.

My experience of a busy London casualty department, and a spell as a Ship's doctor, equipped me better than most. Experience was not needed here, she was dead. She was lying on the pavement, flat on her back, head in a pool of blood and legs characteristically splayed apart. Her eyes were wide and staring though the expression seemed more of wonder than of horror.

"What happened?" I asked inadequately.

"Run over by a horse" said the large, matter of fact ambulance man.

"Sorry, say that again."

"Yes, a bloody runaway horse, hit her fair and square, look at her frame."

He pointed at a mangled piece of aluminium tubing some feet away.

"Didn't do the bloody horse any good either, vet's just shot it."

He gestured to the other gathering down the road. A wave of sadness and of uselessness engulfed me, mingled with a feeling that this was just too unbelievable to be true.

For five years she had never gone out, and the first time she does she is run over by a bolting horse in the centre of a little market town where there are no horses.

A hand touched my sleeve; it was the lady from the Health Food Shop.

"Come with me Doc, I want to show you something."
The ambulance men took Ethel away to the post-mortem room as a favour to the police whose job it was technically. The butcher took the horse away. I was led into her flat.
"The lady at the Post Office said that she screamed 'Elley' just before the horse hit her, I think she thought her old horse had come back for her. Maybe she was right. Here, look here."
She pulled open a large drawer to reveal bottles of pills going back several years, all unopened.
"She didn't believe in pills."
She looked at me pityingly.
"Did you like your shoehorn?"
Not long afterwards, Feb 1975, my father died, from an acute occlusion of the left anterior descending coronary artery. This, as it transpired, turned out to a hereditary weakness. He was 57. I travelled up from the south to help my mother clear out his basement surgery in Beach Road, South Shields.
The smell of damp was strong, a faded print of Landseer's *Monarch of the Glens* was slightly skew-wiff on the mould-covered wall, and it was unutterably gloomy. There were no notes worth the candle, but there was his old microscope, the pestle and mortar, the red, green and brown bottles of non-descript, placebo-laced power, the empty gin bottles, and about five years' worth of the *British Medical Journal*, still in their brown wrappers, piled up on the examination couch. Behind his huge old desk was a little drawer, in which was an open copy of *Tristram Shandy*, and the patient's tatty and rickety chair was placed directly in front of the desk.
My father's funeral at the local crematorium was attended by a larger crowd than the average Sunderland AFC match. So many people I didn't know came up to embrace me (a rare thing for Geordies) and said how much they loved him, but one man stands out in my mind. He sought me out as the crowd was dispersing. He held my hand and looked at me hard.
"Peter, isn't it? And you a doctor, too. Not as good as him, though. Your dad, he was special. He used to listen to you.
Didn't examine you much" (I had worked that one out). "But he listened, and he knew. He always knew, never wrong. Because he always listened, he always knew what mattered."

Howard Thomas

Like Peter Tate and Paul Smith, I too had a fond attachment to cadaver 'S to T' back in 1962/3. George Abouna was our anatomy demonstrator and was very committed to keeping us on the straight and narrow despite some members having a strong propensity for practical jokes. This obviously made a lasting impression on George, who, when I met him several years later in Canada, when he was a distinguished transplant surgeon now without his earlier stutter, suddenly when realizing that I was from his old 'anatomy table' started to stutter again. Clearly not a happy memory!

I also remember Nick Wright who was our group's inspiring pathology demonstrator. My path crossed with Nick again when he became the Dean at the Hammersmith. I was Professor of Medicine at St Mary's, which had merged with Hammersmith to form Imperial College Medical School. Nick was busy buying up the nearby school on behalf of Imperial! Very soon he was Sir Nick.

Mike Marshall, Trevor Lunn and Peter Bore and I opted to do intercalated BScs, leaving the year of 1968 to join the physiology and anatomy departments. Peter Bore and I joined Ivan Jellinek (now Ivan Carrington) to share a flat in Jesmond Dean. I worked with Pavlov pouch dogs in Physiology, Peter worked in Anatomy on thalidomide in rabbits, and Ivan built a Ford Falcon car in our front room. We bought a pressure cooker and lived on the 'control' rabbits from Peter's experiments. Ivan finished his car on Christmas Eve when we jump started the car down Jesmond Hill, to wave him goodbye for Christmas. A few hours later we welcomed him back from the 'Angel of the North', from where he had broken down.

My clinical years, although I had graduated from my BSc and left the year of 1968 to join the year of 1969, were certainly very enjoyable. I particularly remember the month at St Georges (long stay) Psychiatric hospital. The Friday evening patient's dance was a compulsory session overseen by Liz Newton the resident SHO. It is best described as memorable.

I did my obstetric attachment in Hexham; at this time, it was obligatory to deliver a certain number of babies and to do some episiotomy repairs, my first surgical experience.

My final year surgical attachment was at Darlington with Mr K C McKeown. During this attachment I travelled with Mr McKeown to his NHS and private sessions. I assisted him at weekends in the local private hospitals; we had lunch afterwards with the matron of the hospital. McKeown was known for his oesophageal surgery.

On returning to Newcastle my final year medical attachment was to the cardiology unit under Dr Dewar, who was ably assisted by his junior colleague Duncan Newton who gave special attention to collecting the all-essential free fatty acid specimens required for the unit's research. Particularly entertaining were the ward rounds when Dr Dewar regularly asked Duncan for laboratory results which, I suspect, had not been done; there followed a confident citing of some indeterminate results by Duncan, accompanied by a rapid slamming shut of the notes just as Dr Dewar's nose neared the open page. I was only too pleased to stand in for Duncan to allow him time-off to attend 'courses' which I assumed were for his impending MRCP exams but appeared to require a set of golf clubs.

My three months elective was in Baltimore at the Mount Sinai and Johns Hopkins Hospitals. Hopkins was in downtown Baltimore and was a never-ending series of insights into inner city life in the Southern States. On one occasion a man was shot in the Emergency Room by the resident policeman. On another, I was sitting with some other students in the Doctors Residence when two men walked in saying that the television needed taking away for repairing; we never saw it again and no one new anything about a repair.

That year I managed to link my stay in the South with a trip to Expo in Montreal.

I graduated in 1969 and did my first House Job at the RVI with Professors George Smart, John Anderson and David Kerr. In those days at the RVI, we were well cared for and I remember the wonderful conservatory that one passed through on the way to the residences and breakfast.

My second job was with Professors Ivan Johnston, Denis Walder and Brian Flemming with a brief attachment to the plastic surgery unit. In those days, housemen could do minor surgery under supervision; the climax of my surgical career at this time was a single – very difficult but highly successful - appendicectomy.

It might not be surprising that, many years later, when I recounted this episode to Lord Ara Darzi, the Professor of Surgery whose department shared the 10th Floor of St Mary's with my department, he was not impressed.

Immediately after the house jobs I left for an SHO rotation in Glasgow Royal Infirmary. My first job was on the cardiology unit with Professor Veitch Lawrie. On the first night I was shown to the SHO overnight bedroom between the two wards; in those days male and female were separate. In the first week the bleep went off in the middle of the night, the nursing sister appeared at the bedroom door, loaded me up with a bag of kit and a defibrillator, pointed me to a waiting taxi and told me there was a cardiac arrest in Duke Street Hospital, the small hospital 5 minutes away in the Gorbals. Talk about being dropped in at the deep end!

Cardiologists all seem to be characters. The Professor was once told that a patient had jumped from the third floor CCU; his comment was 'did the leads pull off and was the monitor ok'.

I then rotated every few months to the other units before getting my MRCP at the Glasgow College and went to a job as Lecturer in Immunology at the Western Infirmary. Here my life changed in several respects. Two women came into my life. Each year the Pathology staff played cricket against the Scottish National Orchestra where I met Dilys, a viola player. We were introduced by mutual friends and went on to get married. At the same time, I presented a paper at the Medical Research Society on the 'Immunology of the Liver' when I was approached by a short, slightly aggressive lady who at a dinner that evening, grabbed me by the tie and said that 'I was just what she was looking for'. Roddy McSween, the Professor of Pathology at Glasgow, my PhD supervisor, explained that this was Sheila Sherlock, the doyenne of hepatology. Within a few months I was living in a bedsit in Belsize Park Gardens planning my wedding to Dilys and working in Dame Sheila's department at the Royal Free Hospital in Gray's Inn Road. My experience as Lecturer in Medicine was slightly unusual; when I arrived early on my first day, a porter offered to show me to the Academic Department of Medicine. This involved a trip through several corridors, across a roof, up a vertical ladder to a wooden hut on the roof of the hospital. The porter opened the door for me but was reluctant, slightly frightened, to go in. I was greeted by a cheery secretary and shown into the Professor's office.

The welcome was extremely short; Sheila said ‘you’re hepatitis’. The secretary explained that this meant that I was to do some research on viral hepatitis, and I had been allocated the bench between John Summerfield, who was ‘bile salts’, and John Gollan, the Aussie, who was ‘Wilsons’. Because I had done very little clinical medicine and the lectureship was at senior registrar level, I was seconded to look after the professor’s private patients at the Royal Free ‘Liverpool Road’ branch where I was to be ‘brought up to scratch’ by thrice weekly ward rounds with the professor. This was a rude awakening to put it mildly. Luckily, I had come up to standard within a year when the department moved into the new hospital in Hampstead. What a contrast! We had two 30 beds wards, an endoscopy suite and two large laboratory wings, all on the 10th floor overlooking Hampstead Heath. I stayed at the Royal Free for 12 years until I was appointed to a personal chair of Medicine. Research Fellows came from all over the world to work in Sheila Sherlock’s department; I benefited by making many friends and received invitations to visit their countries. I saw most of the world as a consequence.

Each year we had a departmental tennis match at Sheila and her husband, Gerry James’s house, in Hythe. Sheila was always paired with a visiting Australian or South African research fellow who coincidentally was an excellent tennis player; it was no surprise that Sheila won the competition every year.

In 1987 I moved to the Departmental Chair of Medicine at St Mary’s Medical School which eventually merged with Hammersmith and Charing Cross to become Imperial College Medical School. Once again, I moved into a new department on the 10th floor of a new hospital, where I remained for 25 years before retiring in 2011 to Dorset.

On arrival in Dorset, I received a call from Peter Tate, who asked whether I was ‘the Thomas from dissecting table S to T, Newcastle Medical School, 50 years earlier’!

Mike Thompson

An eight-week attachment in Medicine as a final year student proved to be an absolute gem. The consultant was one of those now extinct beings, a general physician but he would occasionally refer a patient for a more specialist opinion. One such patient had a neurological disorder which was, like most it seemed to me, incurable. The referral to John Walton was made with the caveat that if nothing more could be done would he please send the patient back because he was his gardener.

Sir Lancelot Spratt

We had our own Sir Lancelot at the RVI. He had a fearsome reputation. Part of it came from his Tuesday ward rounds where he would grill tremulous students about the patients. The ward rounds were conducted in a manner reminiscent of Richard Gordon's character. The ward was silent (I did hear a pin drop one day) and a sign posted at the entrance to instruct incomers to maintain it. The whole firm was present. The houseman presented the patients. The patients lay to attention in the bed and did not speak until spoken to. The bed sheet was turned down a regulation 14 inches. The sister's stiffly starched apron would crackle as she moved.

Just after the round passed halfway there was a young man with Crohn's disease who had previously had a colectomy as an emergency for a toxic dilatation of the colon. He had been readmitted to have the remaining rectum removed as an elective operation. The senior Registrar was asked about the patient's postoperative progress. He explained that there had been difficulty establishing normal bladder function and that repeated catheterizations had been necessary. With this news, the consultant became very concerned for the patient's welfare saying, "I hope we haven't damaged his nervi erigentes". He then turned to the patient and asked in his booming voice "HAVE YOU HAD AN ERECTION SINCE THE OPERATION?" to which the patient replied "NO SIR" in the manner of a corporal responding to his sergeant major. No titter was heard, and the round moved on.

Had Richard Gordon been present he would have felt he was in familiar territory except, perhaps, that underneath the gruff exterior was an outstanding clinician and a delightful man.

Winning surgical spurs

I had completed a year as Taffy Jones' registrar. Taffy had a long experience of the surgery of portal hypertension and provided a service for the local region. During my year I had done a couple of oesophageal transections under supervision but none "flying solo". I went from that year to a research fellowship in the Department of Surgery at the RVI. My research included a lot of upper GI endoscopy. I was minding my own business early one evening in the endoscopy room, a side room off ward one when Peter Dickinson walked in. He explained that he had a patient with bleeding oesophageal varices who was in trouble and in his view, he needed an oesophageal transection. He had tried to contact the Jones team but to no avail and he knew I had worked on the firm. Would I be willing to do the operation? There really wasn't a choice. There was no-one else around with any experience of this quite major operation and the patient was likely to die without it. I agreed to do the operation.

Peter D said I could use his theatre, theatre main, and he had an anaesthetist. I walked into the theatre and was reminded of its substantial size and, despite refurbishment, on the walls were still the marks of the old gallery for the observers. The patient and surgical team looked pretty small in the middle of this large space.

To add frisson to the operation I had just got started when Peter D and his team came to watch. They stayed for the whole operation. Fortunately, it went without a hitch and the patient did well. I had earned my surgical spurs.

Difficult operations

Some operations are technically challenging, but some are difficult for other reasons.

I had been the senior registrar in the renal transplant unit for seven months and had done one or two transplants with the consultant but none on my own. The consultant went on his summer holiday. What should I do if a transplant became available, I asked? Just do it was the reply.

Sure enough a matching donor and recipient arrived one Saturday. All the arrangements were made there were a few hours to wait. I went for a swim.

The operation took place in the early evening and went well. The kidney functioned from the outset and the postoperative course was uneventful.

The operation was made a bit more difficult because the consultant's holiday started after the 99th transplant had been done on the unit. Kidney disease and transplantation were rarely out of the news locally and nationally so the hundredth had the eyes of the world watching.

Laparoscopic surgery has been an unqualified success but access to deal with major hemorrhage is a bit limited. Laparoscopic splenectomy involves dissecting out the splenic artery and vein and ligating and dividing them. The artery is easy, but the vein is a bit more tricky. The operation is usually performed for ITTP and the thrombocytopaenia is partially corrected with steroids before the operation, so bleeding isn't too much of a problem.

The haematologist appeared on our ward one day with a request for help with such a patient. There were, however, some added complications. The patient was very thrombocytopaenia, did not respond to steroids and was eighteen weeks pregnant. By this stage laparoscopic surgery in pregnancy had been deemed safe but the literature was hardly expansive. There was only one option. Technically the operation went well but the peritoneum and the areolar tissues in the area bruised no matter how careful we were and absorbed some of the available light. Nevertheless, all went smoothly, and the patient was up and about the next day and went home the following day. She subsequently delivered a normal baby without complication. Unfortunately, the press got involved at this stage and the happy event was recorded in the Daily Mail who credited the obstetrician with the splenectomy.

At the back of my mind was the unusual anxiety that if this went wrong, as it had every chance of doing, I would have lost two lives in one operation. There were sighs of relief all round.

Life begins at 40.

One night on call as a senior registrar I was phoned to say that a lady had stabbed herself and was unwell. This was a very rare event in the leafy suburbs of north Bristol in 1976.

On arrival at the hospital, I was greeted by her husband who had explained that she had done it before, and he knew what was going to happen when he heard knives being sharpened in the kitchen.

The patient was 39 and otherwise fit but had evidence of continuing blood loss and some abdominal signs. There were a number of stab wounds above and below the costal margin. The most sophisticated investigation available was a chest x-ray (ultrasound and CT hadn't arrived then) which showed a small amount of pleural fluid. It was difficult to tell whether there was bleeding confined to the chest or that there was also an abdominal injury as two of the abdominal stab wounds raised the distinct possibility of a splenic injury. After some deliberating, I did a laparotomy and a thoracotomy. The knives had missed the spleen and the splenic flexure of the colon by a whisker. The bleeding was coming from the left lung and was easily controlled by a stitch. The patient made an uncomplicated recovery. I saw her in the out-patients department six weeks after her discharge. She was in good spirits and a physical examination was satisfactory. I thought a chest x-ray was in order and, rather than rummaging through her notes I asked her age for the x-ray form. "Oh", she said, "I've just had my birthday. Life begins at 40." I nearly fell off the chair.

Management

I found myself on the Committee to appoint a new manager for the Department of Surgery. One of the candidates, a young man from Glasgow was ushered to the hot seat. He was slightly untidily dressed and his brow moist with perspiration. He was interviewed after which his references were read out. One, from his current Chief Executive was short and to the point. It read "Most NHS managers do not have an original thought in their entire careers: this man is no exception".

Transplant Call

I had never had any interest in being a kidney transplant surgeon but one of my senior registrar attachments included just that. For eighteen months I was on call all day and every day for kidney transplantation in addition to general surgery.

In order to help in the execution of this role I was supplied with a bleep about twice the size of a current TV remote. I was also given a flashing light which worked from the cigarette lighter in the car and had a magnetic base to attach it to the roof in the style of Starsky and Hutch. For some strange reason doctors weren't allowed blue ones so this was red at the front and green at the back. There was a need to move quickly to the donor hospital sometimes as the kidneys could not be removed until the patient was dead but the warm ischaemia time had to be minimized. One such occasion arrived in the late afternoon on a Saturday. The consultant lived just out of town with a long dual carriageway forming part of the route to the hospital. There was a long straight on part of the road followed by a gentle left-hand bend. He had attached his light and drove at speed down the dual carriageway passing a number of cars on the way. As he took the left-hand curve, the centrifugal force acting on the light overcame the centripetal force provided by the magnet, the light crashed to the road and disintegrated. While the bits were recovered all those cars went whizzing past. I returned my light at the end of my appointment unused.

Stan's diet

Howard Young and I were Registrars together on the Plastic Surgery unit at the General hospital in 1970-1. One of the less joyous parts of the job was managing the Burns unit. It could be dramatic. One evening a person was brought in with extensive burns and severe lung damage caused by arson and from which he died the same evening. The unit was flooded with police of senior rank and things moved very quickly including the forensic postmortem that was performed that evening. More often, though, events were much less dramatic.

With extensive burns care and recovery was a slow process during which nutrition could be a problem. Stan was a patient in just this position. His body mass and his plasma albumin were both low and need to be corrected. Although his digestive tract was functioning his appetite was poor.

The hospital chef came to the ward to see Stan. The chef offered to make Stan whatever he wanted. We all supposed he would choose something like a nice steak or a roast meal but no.

After questioning the surprisingly good offer he made his choice. It was to be a plate of raw tripe. We couldn't believe it. However, he ate a plate piled high with raw tripe twice a day from then on, the whole lot. And sure enough, his albumin rose, his weight increased, his wounds healed, and he was eventually discharged.

Wells Cottage Hospital

With my appointment to a consultant's post in Bristol came a fortnightly session at the Wells Cottage Hospital, about an hour's drive away. The session alternated between an out-patient clinic and an operating list. There was a sister in charge of each function. To call them departments would be stretching matters a bit.

The service was hugely appreciated by the patients. They had a consultant opinion on their doorstep and without a huge waiting list. The GPs ran a 24-hour casualty service so avoiding the trip to Bristol. On one occasion an elderly man with bad COAD came into the consulting room short of breath just walking on the flat. He needed a hernia repair. When I explained to him the need to come to Bristol for his hernia repair because of his chest he would have none of it: he wanted his operation to be done in Wells. It took some time to convince him such was the attraction of the local service.

There also happened to be a good shoe-shop in Wells and it was possible to park outside of it. I could exchange my worn-out shoes for the same model easily. It closed at 5.30. To finish the clinic by that time was difficult until I discovered how.

The sister gave me the referral letter, so I knew what was wrong with the patient before they came in. The consulting room was quite large with the desk on the far side from the door and the examination couch in between.

If time was short it was possible to greet the patient coming into the room and, if appropriate, escort them directly to the couch thus avoiding the time-consuming move to and from the patient's chair. All the normal pleasantries and standards were preserved but time was not wasted.

Operating was in an old theatre with a part glass roof, similar to the one at Walker Park hospital. The theatre window faced west so it was nice and sunny. If it got too hot the windows were opened. There was a sister in charge who doubled as the sister on the male ward.

The patient's GP came to assist and one of them gave the anaesthetics. They also provided such post-operative care as was required. Wound infection was unheard of. The process was well established and efficient but had the odd wrinkle. I discovered, after some years, that the patients were given a couple of glycerin suppositories on arrival at the hospital to empty the bowels, a practice which had long ceased elsewhere.

There was only one serious problem and that was a young man with a hernia who went into intense laryngospasm during intubation and went a bit blue. The anaesthetist was struggling, and I was poised to do a tracheotomy when his airway opened up and all was well.

The journey to Wells went through some lovely countryside and was a joy in summer. In winter crossing two sets of hills could be hazardous if snowy. Rain plagues the south west more than snow in the winter. I was driving back to Bristol after the clinic one dark winter's evening with lashing rain when my bleep sounded (this was before mobile phones) so I stopped at a phone box. In the dark I stepped straight into a deep puddle only to find several of the windows were missing, there was no light, and the rain and wind were lashing the inside of the box. Fortunately, the phone was working, and I had the appropriate coin. Eventually I got through to the physician trying to find me. His first words were "Oh, hello, Mike, it's not urgent".

Eventually, the operating and then the consulting was stopped. The hospital has been converted into apartments. The patients now have to journey further but at least they will be spared two suppositories.

The King's pneumonectomy

On Sunday, September 23rd, 1951 King George V1th underwent a pneumonectomy. The surgeon was Sir Clement Price-Thomas.

The story goes that Price-Thomas knew that his royal patient should be treated exactly the same as any other patient, on the Health service or privately. The only difference was that the operation was undertaken at Buckingham Palace. However, everything else was the same.

The equipment to be used was that in daily use at the Westminster Hospital and the theatre nurses those who regularly worked with Price-Thomas at the Westminster Hospital. The assistants were also from the hospital, Charles Drew and Peter Jones. They had to live at the palace for the King's post-operative care. The King did well.

One afternoon I received a phone call from the Medical Director of the London Clinic. It was to ask if I would be willing to undertake a laparoscopic cholecystectomy on one of the Arab leaders.
Apparently, the reason for the request was some evidence that the patient might have stones in his common bile duct. At that time, we were one of few centres in the country able to deal with bile duct stones laparoscopically. The operation requires a significant amount of specialist equipment and a theatre staff who know how it works.
I remembered the story of the King's pneumonectomy. I, therefore, said I would be happy to help but the patient would have to come to Bristol because we couldn't take all the equipment and staff to London and I wouldn't use any equipment in London as it would have to be borrowed. I also asked our department manager if we could do this. "Of course," was his reply, "we'll clear a ward". (Quite how he thought he could do that escaped me.)
After a few days the London "fixer" rang back and declined my offer. He had found a surgeon who was prepared to go to London. The patient did well.

Stuart Walton

A few memories

Whilst I was in Nairobi, we had a visit from my old boss in Newcastle, John Lawson, an internationally recognised expert on the treatment of Vesicovaginal fistula. Naturally we put on a special case for him to operate which he did with great aplomb before flying off to Tanzania. I joined him for a conference in Moshi and his first words were asking about the patient he had left behind. I replied that she was well after we cut the sutures that had been blocking both her ureters! ----

I was on call and just before I left for home, I called in on the Labour Ward. The Midwife said that my registrar was delivering a breech, so I decided to stay in the coffee room until he had finished. Within 5 minutes I was called in to find the breech was hanging out 'FACE TO PUBES'. Not the accepted way of delivering! I took over and despite trying to get my hands in to try and turn the baby manually I was having great difficulty in working out how to get the baby out and I could see that the cord had stopped pulsating. I asked for a pair of Neville Barnes forceps, placed them directly on to the baby's head and pulled. The baby was successfully delivered almost immediately. When I got back to the coffee room, I recounted this to my Senior Registrar for which he replied that he had read somewhere that that was the correct way to deliver the baby stuck like that. Another case of "making it up as you go along" and finding you've done the right thing. -----

Dryburn Hospital was built on the basis of a central corridor with wards coming off along its Path and the corridor was uphill. The Labour Ward was halfway up, and the theatres were at the top. No problem usually but when faced with a prolapsed cord in Labour in the middle of visiting hour could prove little embarrassing.

Trundling up the corridor at full speed with the patient in the knee chest position and you endeavouring to keep the cord of the oncoming head with your two fingers was not the most edifying sight for visitors in the same corridor. Thankfully it only happened once! Mike Marshall was surgical registrar at the same time, and I am sure he must have had similar experiences.

That place up the road (not the RVI)

In Newcastle, the General Hospital in the 60s did not have the status of a "Teaching Hospital", but it was integral in providing both medical care and education in the city. Indeed, some of the predominant disciplines were housed here e.g., Radiotherapy, Neurology and Neurosurgery, and many supplicant services carried as much weight as those "down the road" e.g., Urology and Cardiology.

For our year in 1965, at the completion of our Preclinical years, the first real exposure to medicine and surgery was the summer holiday secondment to the General. I was assigned to the Casualty Department (not called A&E then) and it was there that I became acquainted with a wealth of acute medicine and surgery but also learning the rudiments of cleaning and stitching wounds which included the important skill of knot tying. Upstairs Mr Alf Petty had established an excellent acute surgical unit dealing with chest injuries and other major trauma not the domain of orthopaedic and neurosurgeons. My next experience was on the medical wards 3&4, under the supervision of Christo Strang specialising in pulmonary disease (the 'pink puffers' and 'blue bloaters') and I established a rudimentary knowledge in clinical diagnosis and management to be developed later in our subsequent years of lectures and clinical attachments. The wards had a long-lasting effect on me as I chose that Unit for my Final Year medical attachment and my House Job on qualification. The hospital provided a friendly atmosphere away from the academic milieu we found in the RVI and this probably determined my choice of institution for my early postgraduate career.

I was appointed House Officer to the Strang Unit dividing my 6 months into 3 equal positions on Male, Female and Geriatric Wards with the other 2 House Officers (the latter Ward was under the guidance of Mike Hall who later became one of the first Professors of Geriatric Medicine).

We had one Registrar (Mike Lye, later the Prof of Geriatric Medicine in Liverpool), 2 SHOs and 2 Ward Sisters who very often had more clinical knowledge than all the doctors combined.

All junior doctors were housed in the 'Mess' at the top of the hospital and there was a sense of belonging to the Organisation one rarely sees today.

One of the sayings then was that the worst times for patients to have a heart attack or other medical emergency were Thursday and Sunday evenings at 7 pm as they coincided with everyone downing tools and congregating in the Mess to see "Top of the Pops" and "Rowan & Martin's Laugh In" respectively! Across the road from the hospital was a Bowling Alley and the '69 Club' and we discovered early on that our bleeps worked very well from there. There was an abundance of characters at the hospital and not just the consultants. Our Orderly, Eric, had been a Head Waiter at the Ritz in London and this had considerable advantages when we were called out at 2am for a cardiac arrest. When it became obvious that the patient was either going to make it or not, Mike Lye would gesture to Eric who then disappeared. Half an hour later after clearing up, we were met in the office with a wealth of open sandwiches (often cucumber) and cakes, we never asked as to where they had been sourced. Word 21 was the Private Wing, and we were often asked to perform routine testing for Christo. My most notable attendance was to Lord Lambton (later scandalised for his forays with the 'second profession') although I never asked as to the medical condition for which he was in! My second 6 months was spent on the Surgical Side and I was Houseman to Mr Raoul Piachaud, a very private and upright man who was the perfect foil to his colleague, Mr Dudfield Rose. Mr Piachaud was a "General Surgeon" in all aspects of the word, and it was not unusual to have a thyroidectomy, a thoracotomy and a bowel resection all on the same list. When confronted with an abdomen full of adhesions and fibrous tissue he constantly uttered "Oh dear, we should never have started!" However, within 45 minutes he had performed an immaculate Total Gastrectomy. Dudfield Rose was the antithesis of this. His speciality of gall bladder surgery was legendary and, using a Rio Branco Incision he could perform a cholecystectomy in 15-20 minutes skin to skin! The only downside was that further work was required to repair the incisional hernia created by this 'mega flap incision'! The Unit consisted of two Consultants, one Registrar, one SHO and me. As the Unit was always on call for their patients, it meant at times that I could be on for 16 continuous days and nights while the SHO was on holiday. It was a time when we experienced a quantity as well as a quality of experience and I don't think I suffered as a result. Additional to other duties I was assigned a Minor Surgical Outpatient clinic taking off sebaceous cysts, skin tags and lassoing piles. All these experiences helped in my development to a surgical orientated career in O&G.

I will remember with fondness the House Year at the NGH. The clinical medical and surgical experiences obtained were exceptional, the camaraderie of the "Mess" unforgettable and the characters memorable. Somehow, we expected to be worked hard and didn't complain about hours worked. The (?) princely salary of £1100 per annum was a damn sight better than the student grant we had lived on for the previous 5 years and we probably didn't get a lot of opportunity to spend it anyway. It kept us in beer, cigarettes and 10 pin Bowling. It was no surprise that, having chosen O&G as a career, I applied for an SHO post at the General at the conclusion of my House Year. During my stint as SHO in O&G during one of Dorothea Kerslake's Gynae clinics, the registrar came in and said there was a lady from Gateshead aged 40 with 5 children wanting a sterilisation. Dorothea immediately retorted "Sterilise every bugger from Gateshead!" Little did she know that was my hometown!

Howard Young. (contributed by Louise Young)
Snippets

1. During my time as a young registrar. A patient came in having a very nasty vaginal discharge. They admitted her and took her to surgery. On examining her there was obviously something lodged high up inside, carefully I pulled out what turned out to be a rolled up poster of Elvis Presley! It had been there for near enough two years!
2. Surgeons all wear clogs whilst operating. This particular Aberdeen surgeon I worked with had noticed someone had been using his clogs. So, he decided to write wee note on his right shoe. Saying "I've got veruccas". On his return the next day, he noticed another written note on his left shoe. It said, "So have I".
3. In Newcastle RVI a Chinese lady was admitted to the ward. It was late in the day and everyone had put in what they had wanted to eat for their evening meal. The sister in charge of the ward took upon herself to choose something the lady would like. At dinner time dishing out the meal the ward sister put down a plate in front of this lady and bent over whispering. (Geordie accent required here) "I got you a nice piece of rice puddin".

Thanks to Pete Irvin for the exam papers. I suspect we all still get the chills looking at them.

December, 1964 | *Time—Three Hours*

UNIVERSITY OF NEWCASTLE UPON TYNE

Stage I Examination for the Degrees of Bachelor of Medicine and Bachelor of Surgery.

PAPER I

Answer **FOUR** questions.

Illustrate your answers, as far as possible, with diagrams.

The answer to each question must be written in a separate book.
Write the number of the question on the cover of the answer book.

1. Describe the conducting system in the heart and discuss the factors which control the heart rate.

2. Describe the blood supply of the stomach and the microanatomy of the gastric glands. Give an account of the factors controlling gastric secretion.

3. What methods are available for the study of the human cerebral cortex? What information has been gained by these methods about the sensory functions of the cortex?

4. Describe the structural organisation of bone and discuss the metabolism of its mineral content.

5. Describe the structure of the mammary gland, with a brief note on its lymphatic drainage. Describe the hormonal control of mammary development and lactation.

December, 1964 | *Time—Three Hours*

UNIVERSITY OF NEWCASTLE UPON TYNE

Stage I Examination for the Degrees of Bachelor of Medicine and Bachelor of Surgery.

PAPER II

Answer **FOUR** questions.

Illustrate your answers, as far as possible, with diagrams.

The answer to each question must be written in a separate book.
Write the number of the question on the cover of the answer book.

1. What is the organisation of education in Newcastle at the present time? How is education influenced by health?

2. Describe, with experimental evidence, current concepts of the reabsorption of water from renal tubular fluid in the mammalian kidney. Indicate in detail how far the structure of the nephron appears to correlate with these concepts.

3. Discuss the functional anatomy of the lower respiratory tract (secondary bronchi to alveoli). Give an account of the early and late reactions of the body to a lack of oxygen in the air breathed.

4. Give an account of the microanatomy of the liver and describe the role of this organ in the digestion, absorption and metabolism of lipids.

5. Discuss the structural and functional aspects of the composition and circulation of tissue (interstitial) fluid.

June, 1965 *Time—Three Hours*

UNIVERSITY OF NEWCASTLE UPON TYNE

Stage II Examination for the Degrees of Bachelor of Medicine and Bachelor of Surgery

PAPER I

Answer **ALL** the questions.

SECTION A.

The answer to the questions in this section must be written in the book marked A.

1. Differentiate between bacteraemia, septicaemia and pyaemia. Describe in detail the technique of blood culture including the subsequent laboratory procedures involved in a case of staphylococcal septicaemia.

2. Discuss the bacteriological diagnosis, epidemiology and prevention of tetanus.

3. Write notes on any five of the following:
   - (a) Log phase of bacterial growth
   - (b) Bacterial spores
   - (c) Bacterial reproduction
   - (d) Agglutination
   - (e) Small-pox immunisation
   - (f) Haemagglutination
   - (g) Lancefield grouping

SECTION B.

The answer to question 4 in this section must be written in the book marked B.

The answer to questions 5 and 6 must be written as indicated on the separate question papers provided and these must be handed to the invigilator at the end of the examination.

4. What does the term *hypertrophy* mean? Discuss the factors involved in its production by reference to examples from man.

June, 1965 *Time—Three Hours*

UNIVERSITY OF NEWCASTLE UPON TYNE

Stage II Examination for the Degrees of Bachelor of Medicine and Bachelor of Surgery

PAPER II

Answer **SIX** questions, of which **FIVE** must be chosen from Sections A and B.

The answers to questions in Section A must be written in the book marked A.
The answers to questions in Section B must be written in the book marked B.
The answer to the question in Section C must be written in the book marked C.

Candidates are requested to write the numbers of the questions they have attempted on the cover of each answer book in the order in which they appear in it.

SECTION A.

1. Discuss the biochemical laboratory investigations carried out on patients suffering from intestinal malabsorption.

2. Discuss the origin and fate of bilirubin.

3. Discuss the ways in which the maintenance of the cell depends upon its energy supply.

SECTION B.

4. Give an account of the pharmacological actions of the digitalis glycosides. Discuss briefly their main therapeutic uses and the effects of overdosage.

5. Discuss the principles involved in the absorption, distribution, metabolism and excretion of drugs. Illustrate your answer by reference to particular drugs.

6. Give an account of the two main groups of analgesics. Discuss the relative advantages and disadvantages of those drugs which you mention.

SECTION C.

7. What is meant by the following?
   - (a) Ionising radiation dosemeter
   - (b) Industrial deafness
   - (c) Maximum Allowable Concentration
   - (d) Frequency distribution
   - (e) Statistical correlation

May, 1967 *Time—Two Hours.*

Final Examination for the Degrees of Bachelor of Medicine and Bachelor of Surgery (Part I)

(New Regulations)

PAPER II

Answer **ONE** question from each section

The answer to the question in Section A must be written in the book marked A.
The answer to the question in Section B must be written in the book marked B.
The answer to the question in Section C must be written in the book marked C.

Candidates must write the number of the question they have attempted on the cover of each answer book.

SECTION A.

1. Discuss the value of chromosome examination in the diagnosis of disease.

2. Discuss the value of defining vulnerable or 'high risk' groups in relation to certain disorders; mention specific examples in your discussion.

3. Two days after a major abdominal operation a patient is found to be oliguric. Give an account of the possible causes and indicate the investigations you would undertake and treatment you would institute.

4. What is the biological value of pain to the individual? Illustrate how a knowledge of the ways in which pain is produced can help in the diagnosis of 'the acute abdomen' in childhood.

(TURN OVER

SECTION B.

5. Write an essay on drug dependence.

6. Discuss the diagnosis and management of cardiac arrest.

7. Write an essay on "The use of antiseptics in 1967."

8. Discuss growth in childhood with particular reference to puberty and adolescence.

SECTION C.

9. Give an account of the secretion of hormones during a normal menstrual cycle. What action would you take if a patient presented with amenorrhœa?

10. Which vitamins are mothers advised to give young children regularly in this country at the present time? What specific effects on the tissues do they produce? Describe the clinical picture which may result from deficiency of *one* of these vitamins.

11. Discuss pyrexia of uncertain origin.

12 Enumerate the injuries to the upper limb which commonly result from a fall on the outstretched hand. Take one of these and discuss it in detail, including possible complications, prognosis and treatment.

Final Examination for the Degrees of Bachelor of Medicine and Bachelor of Surgery (Part I)

(New Regulations)

PAPER III

Answer **ONE** question from each section

The answer to the question in Section A must be written in the book marked A.
The answer to the question in Section B must be written in the book marked B.
The answer to the question in Section C must be written in the book marked C.

Candidates must write the number of the question they have attempted on the cover of each answer book.

SECTION A.

1. Describe the position and main relations of the pituitary gland. Explain the symptoms and signs that may be associated with an expanding (non-secretory) tumour of the pituitary.

2. Screening procedures (quick and approximate methods of picking out those who probably have a disorder, especially a latent one, from those who probably do not) may be one way of controlling certain diseases. What criteria determine the suitability of a screening procedure for general use?

3. Discuss the epidemiology of accidents and their prevention.

4. Describe the ill health for which the β-hæmolytic streptococcus may be responsible and outline the steps that can be taken to minimise the effects of these organisms.

(TURN OVER

SECTION B.

5. Discuss the use of liver function tests in distinguishing between the various types of jaundice.

6. Discuss the significance of anorexia as a psychiatric symptom.

7. Describe the methods at present available for family limitation.

8. You are a family doctor and a 'blue baby' (Fallot's tetralogy) is born into your practice. Describe your management of the case over the next ten years.

SECTION C.

9. Children are immunised against a number of infectious diseases. Write an account of the programme of immunisation and state the nature of the preparation used for each disease.

10. What types of urticaria do you know of? Discuss three of these in detail.

11. Discuss the diagnosis and management of facial paralysis.

12. Discuss the ætiology, clinical features and management of Parkinson's disease.

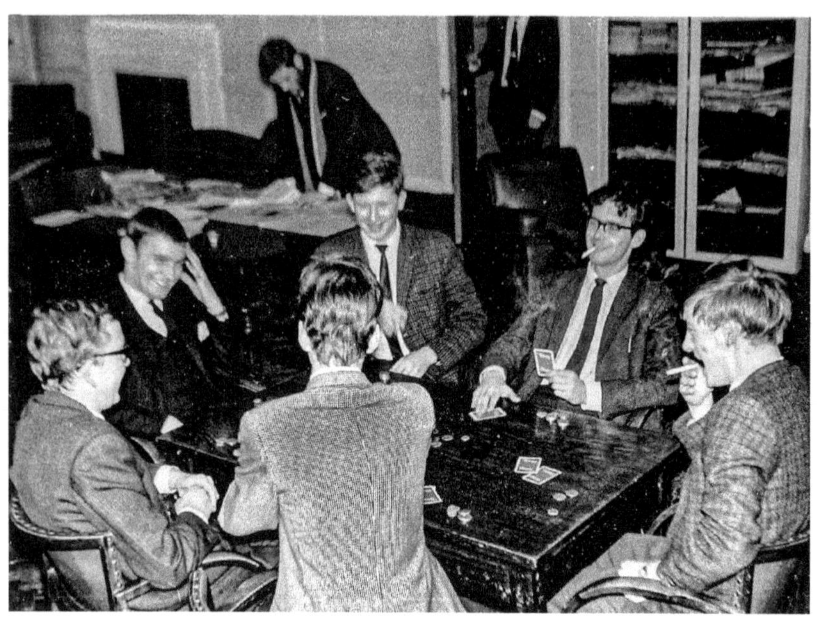

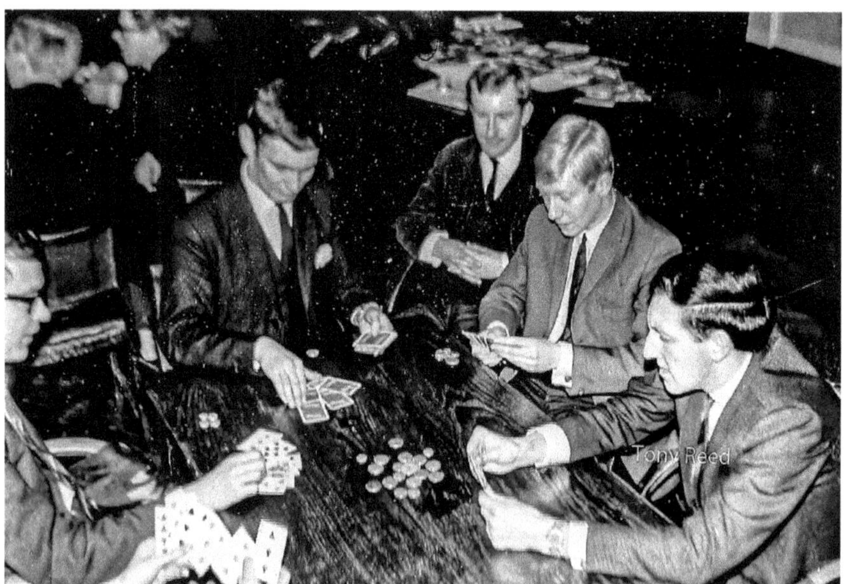

Seven card stud in the common Room. 1964

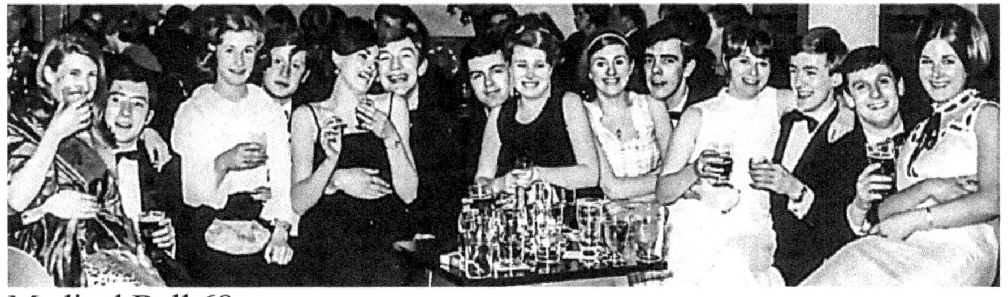
Medical Ball 68

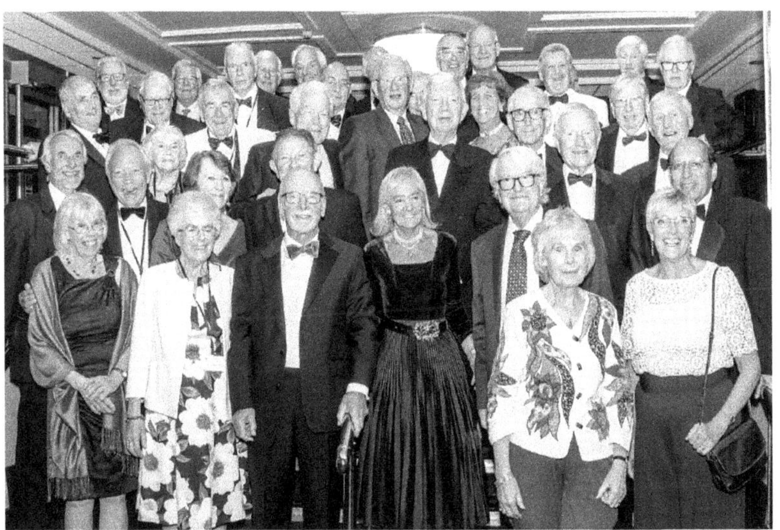
In 2018 At the 50 year reunion.

www.ingramcontent.com/pod-product-compliance
Ingram Content Group UK Ltd.
Pitfield, Milton Keynes, MK11 3LW, UK
UKHW022025190726
13853UKWH00005B/2115

9 798734 520345